"Congratulations on an extremely informative, accurate and readable book on a timely subject vital to millions of women. I know of no other source which combines a discussion of the most advanced medical and pharmacological treatments with alternative therapies, nutrition advice and psychological counseling."

—Burton V. Caldwell, M.D., Ph.D.
Metabolism Associates

The Taking Charge of Menopause
WORKBOOK

Robert M. Dosh, Ph.D.

Susan N. Fukushima, M.D.

Jane E. Lewis, Ph.D.

Robert L. Ross, M.D.

Lynne A. Steinman, Ph.D.

NEW HARBINGER PUBLICATIONS

Publisher's Note

This publication is designed to provide accurate and authoritative information in regard to the subject matter covered. It is sold with the understanding that the publisher is not engaged in rendering psychological, financial, legal, or other professional services. If expert assistance or counseling is needed, the services of a competent professional should be sought.

Copyright © 1997 by Robert M. Dosh, Ph.D., Susan N. Fukushima, M.D., Jane E. Lewis, Ph.D., Robert L. Ross, M.D., and Lynne A. Steinman, Ph.D.
New Harbinger Publications, Inc.
5674 Shattuck Avenue
Oakland, CA 94609

ISBN Paperback 1-57224-060-1

Distributed in U.S.A. by Publishers Group West; in Canada by Raincoast Books; in Great Britain by Airlift Book Company, Ltd.; in South Africa by Real Books, Ltd.; in Australia by Boobook; in New Zealand by Tandem Press.

Edited by Farrin Alyse Jacobs
Text Design by Michele Waters
Cover Design by SHELBY DESIGNS & ILLUSTRATES

Printed in the United States on recycled paper.

10 9 8 7 6 5 4 3 2 1

Contents

Acknowledgments

We would like to acknowledge our spouses and families for providing the support, time, and space to complete this book. We would also like to thank Dr. Stephen M. Lieb and Lidia Rubenstein for their time and energy in reading our book and providing useful suggestions. Finally, we would like to thank Laura Young, our Administrative Assistant, who so tirelessly worked on the many drafts of our book.

Introduction

Menopause, a word derived from two Greek words meaning, "month," and "cessation," is a life transition that currently affects millions of American women, ranging in age from forty-five to fifty-four. With the average life expectancy of women approaching eighty years, 20 percent of the population will live more than a third of their lives in postmenopause. At the present time, there are forty million women who are menopausal. Over the next decade, an additional twenty million women will go through menopause.

While your mother may have talked to you about menstruation and childbirth, the other two biological transitions in the lives of women, she did not usually talk about or prepare you for menopause. Thus, menopause has often been anticipated with anxiety and dread. It has been associated with both frightening and embarrassing symptoms, and with the end of a woman's sexuality. It has frequently been regarded as marking the passage into old age. This book will help you understand that menopause is a natural biological transition; it is not a disease and does not need to be perceived negatively. If you know more about this transition, you can communicate with your physician and make your own health care choices in order to minimize uncomfortable changes that might arise during menopause. With this knowledge, you can continue to lead a productive and vital life.

What Is Menopause?

Menopause, strictly defined, refers to the last menstrual period and is retroactively identified when one year has passed since that menstrual period. However, most people use the term to encompass the biological changes that span a period of about ten to fifteen years, when the ovaries gradually stop producing eggs and hormones. The medical term for this period is *climacteric* from the Greek *klima* (the ladder). Because of its common usage, this book will refer to the climacteric as menopause. During this time, periods are often erratic and infrequent, menopausal changes appear, and fertility is impaired.

Below is a table of terms often used when discussing menopause.

Table 1
Terms to Know About Menopause

Perimenopause	The time from the onset of hormonal and menstrual changes to one year into menopause
The Menopause	The final menstrual period
Postmenopause	The time after menopause
Climacteric	The period when the ovaries stop producing eggs and hormones, commonly referred to as menopause

Viewing Menopause As a Natural Biological Transition

This book approaches the subject of menopause with a focus on *wellness*. The National Wellness Institute defines wellness as "an active process of becoming aware of and making choices toward a more successful existence."

In moving toward wellness, you can begin by accepting that the physical changes happening to your body are a natural biological transition. You can focus on feeling good, as opposed to seeing menopause as a disease or as creating illness. Many women use this time to evaluate and reassess life choices. Further, menopause can be a time to work on achieving a sense of life balance and greater self-esteem, and creating new areas of life fulfillment.

Throughout this book, you will be encouraged to make informed decisions about your health and lifestyle. The decisions you make need to be the ones that are right for you, even if they are not the popular ones. It is important to give yourself the right to change a decision if further information becomes available to warrant it.

Making choices results in an increased sense of personal control and emotional well-being. In order to make the best choices possible, it is essential to have the information necessary for interacting in a collaborative way with your health care providers. The purpose of this book is to provide you with this information so you can

- Take charge of your health

- Formulate your own individual plan to deal with the changes you experience during menopause

How to Use This Book

This book is designed to be read in small segments so that you can pick it up and put it down as your time permits and your interests change. It is an invaluable guide that you can refer to throughout the perimenopausal years, as well as during the early postmenopausal years. The checklists, exercises, and other graphic aids in this book have been specifically designed to help you gather information so that you can take charge of this transition. Each chapter focuses on a specific area. In the last chapter ("Putting It All Together"), you are given the materials that will allow you to make informed decisions and design your own personalized plan to optimize your experience of menopause.

Although this book is primarily directed toward women experiencing menopause, it is hoped that it will also appeal to family members and to medical and mental health professionals who are treating perimenopausal and menopausal women.

Below are a list of questions commonly asked about menopause. Place a check mark next to any that are of interest to you. After each question, the chapter numbers in which you will find the answers are listed.

General

_____ 1. Am I menopausal? (2)

_____ 2. Are there any tests that will tell if I'm menopausal? (2)

_____ 3. At what age does menopause occur? (2)

Medical

_____ 4. What medical tests should a menopausal woman have, and how often? (appendix A)

_____ 5. Do I still need to have pelvic exams and Pap smears after menopause? (appendix A)

_____ 6. What if I have irregular bleeding? (3, 5)

_____ 7. Will walking prevent osteoporosis? (8)

_____ 8. Can vitamins and minerals help prevent heart disease? Osteoporosis? (8)

_____ 9. Will sex change at menopause? (3, 9)

_____ 10. What can I do about sexual problems because of vaginal dryness? (3, 6, 7)

_____ 11. What are Kegel exercises? (4)

_____ 12. When can I stop using birth control? (9)

_____ 13. Sometimes, when I cough or laugh, I'll lose a little urine. Is that normal? What can I do about it? (4, 6)

_____ 14. When is a hysterectomy necessary? (5)

_____ 15. I've had a hysterectomy. How will menopause differ for me? (5)

Hormone Replacement Therapy

_____ 16. Should I take estrogen? (6)

_____ 17. Do I have to take progesterone if I take estrogen? (6)

_____ 18. If I decide to take hormones, how long will I have to take them? (6)

_____ 19. Which is better—the estrogen pill or the patch? (6)

_____ 20. If I use hormones, will my period start again? (6)

_____ 21. Is there anything besides hormones that can help with hot flashes? (3, 6, 7)

_____ 22. If I take HRT, do I need to worry about osteoporosis and heart disease? (4, 6)

_____ 23. Should I still take estrogen if cancer is in my family? (6)

_____ 24. Will estrogen prevent heart disease? (4, 6)

Psychological/Interpersonal

_____ 25. Will I get depressed or have mood swings when I'm menopausal? (10)

_____ 26. What can I do about irritability and depression? (10, 11)

_____ 27. What are the more common psychological/emotional problems during the menopausal years? (10)

_____ 28. Do you have any tips on coping with stress? (12)

_____ 29. I need some help communicating with my doctor. What can I do? (15)

_____ 30. My husband thinks hot flashes are in my head. What can I tell him? (14)

_____ 31. Do men go through menopause? (14)

Evaluating New Research

As medical research is constantly producing new knowledge, studies cited today may be obsolete in six months. Thus, keeping abreast of current research is critical. Many articles in newspapers or magazines that attract attention are written from a sensationalist point of view. In order to get beyond the sensationalism and truly evaluate the content of these articles, it is helpful to know how research is conducted. Please refer to appendix D for more specific information about research and the scientific method of conducting studies.

1

The History, Politics, and Culture of Menopause

This chapter will cover

- A historical review of menopause

- A brief review of cross-cultural studies

- The politics of menopause and women's health in the United States

Historical Review

From the time at which the term was first used, up to the 1960s, menopause was perceived as a disease and thought to cause a multitude of symptoms and illnesses, ranging from diarrhea to diabetes. Well into the 1900s, thousands of women were committed to mental institutions, diagnosed as having a mental disease called "involutional melancholia," which was thought to be related to menopause. Some physicians characterized menopausal women as "peevish," or "quarrelsome and obstinate."

It is understandable then why women have anticipated menopause with fear and apprehension. One of the challenges facing women today is to change this negative image of menopause. Instead of associating it with old age, sickness, and loss of sexuality and attractiveness, women are beginning to look at menopause as a positive natural event. They are dispelling the myth of it being a deficiency disease, or a medical or psychological crisis.

Cross-Cultural Studies

Cross-cultural studies support the idea that menopause can be a positive life event. There are cultures in the world where menopause is viewed favorably. In such cultures there are often fewer physical complaints associated with the cessation of menstruation when compared to those cultures in which menopause is viewed negatively.

For example, a study of Indian women of the Rajput caste found no evidence of the depression or other negative changes associated with menopause that have frequently been reported elsewhere. The researchers felt that this was because, after menopause, previously veiled and secluded women in that caste are given access to many of the activities formerly reserved only for men. Thus, for them menopause means greater status and freedom. This is also the case in other non-Western cultures where postmenopausal women encounter culturally sanctioned role changes that either increase their status or decrease their burdens.

Even in the West there are groups that are more accepting of menopause. For example, Amish women often view menopause as a natural part of life, and therefore, stay active, confront changes positively, and even maintain a sense of humor about it.

Most cross-cultural studies reveal that the status of postmenopausal women is increased in cultures where there are

- Strong ties to the extended family system
- Social systems that extol strong mother-child relationships and reproduction
- Well-defined grandmother and mother-in-law roles
- Extensive menstrual taboos
- Respect and reverence for age

In contrast, having a youth-oriented culture increases the potential for problems during menopause. What you can learn from other cultures is that the presence of a clearly defined role, positive status for postmenopausal women, and important life tasks beyond childrearing years are significant factors determining the way women react to menopause.

Politics of Menopause and Women's Health

Another reason for the negative images and messages surrounding menopause has been women's limited political power within the medical and research communities, as well as within society as a whole. Until fairly recently, most physicians were men. Women who consulted physicians about physical complaints or symptoms occurring during menopause were often patronized by male doctors, or dismissed as "hysterical."

Also until recently, studies about diseases and their treatments often did not include women. Much of the information about the causes, treatments, and prevention of illness comes from studies conducted primarily with men and therefore may not be applicable for specific health problems as they affect women.

In a study conducted in 1990 by the U.S. General Accounting Office, only 13.5 percent of the budget of the National Institutes of Health (NIH) was used for research related to diseases or health concerns unique to women. This fact is especially significant since women are responsible for two-thirds of all health care dollars spent, suffer greater disability, and have poorer health outcomes from chronic illnesses than do men.

Fortunately, the federal government has recently created new policies, programs, and offices to deal with women's health care issues in unprecedented ways. Further, changes in women's roles in both the workplace and the home have resulted in greater access to information, and an expectation that women's concerns will be taken more seriously than they have been in the past.

As a result of all of these factors, women now have greater representation within medical research, experience more responsiveness from the medical profession, and have their concerns taken more seriously by society at large. Consequently, they are becoming more active participants in their own health care management.

Summary

- Women of today are changing the negative image of menopause.

- Views about menopause vary with cultures.

- Women now have more political power and leverage within the medical profession and in medical research.

- Women are becoming more active participants in their own health care management.

2

The Biology of Menopause

If you understand the normal menstrual cycle and how the female reproductive system works before menopause, it will be easier to understand why menopause occurs. This chapter will

- Review the biology of the normal menstrual cycle
- Discuss changes that occur in the menstrual cycle during perimenopause

You will also find out about:

- When menopause occurs
- Premature menopause
- Late menopause
- How to determine whether you are perimenopausal

Why Does Menopause Occur?

The menstrual cycle is dependent on the endocrine system and hormones. The endocrine system is a group of glands located throughout the body that produce chemicals called *hormones*. These hormones travel through the body via the blood stream and act as messengers, telling specific organs how to behave.

In the reproductive system, three glands are important: the *hypothalamus*, the *pituitary*, and the *ovaries*. The hypothalamus and the pituitary are located in your brain; the ovaries are on either side of your uterus. The hypothalamus links the brain to the endocrine system and orchestrates the menstrual cycle through its action on the pituitary.

The menstrual cycle lasts an average of twenty-eight days. During the first fourteen days of the cycle, known as the *follicular phase*, (with day one defined as the first day of menstrual bleeding) the hypothalamus sends signals to the pituitary to release *follicle stimulating hormone* (FSH). FSH stimulates several egg cells, or follicles, within the ovaries to grow. As the follicles develop, they produce *estrogen,* which causes the lining of the uterus to thicken and thereby prepares the uterus for pregnancy.

During each menstrual cycle, one follicle dominates and continues to grow while the others die. Around the fourteenth day of the cycle, the hypothalamus sends another message to the pituitary telling it to secrete *luteinizing hormone* (LH). LH causes the dominant follicle to be released from the ovary and to travel to the *fallopian tube* where it may or may not be fertilized. This is known as *ovulation*.

At the previous site of the follicle, the adjacent cells multiply and connect to each other to form the corpus luteum (yellow body). The corpus luteum continues to produce estrogen in much lower levels but also begins producing large amounts of a second hormone, *progesterone*. Progesterone stimulates cells in the uterine lining to secrete nutrients that will nourish the egg if it becomes fertilized. If the egg does not become fertilized, the corpus luteum gets smaller and stops secreting progesterone and estrogen. Without these hormones, the cells of the uterine lining die and, along with blood and some mucus, form the menstrual flow.

Before menstruation begins, the low levels of estrogen and progesterone alert the hypothalamus to start the cycle again. The hypothalamus again sends its messengers to the pituitary and the cycle begins again.

The ovary has about two million eggs at birth. By the time girls begin to menstruate, there are only about seventy-five thousand left. After puberty, eight to ten eggs grow each month. Usually only one of them will mature.

About ten years before the menopause, the ovaries start running out of eggs, fertility decreases, estrogen production decreases, and menstrual cycles may become abnormal. The pituitary continues to release FSH and LH in the hope of stimulating the ovary, so FSH and LH levels rise. As menopause draws nearer, ovulation stops and so does progesterone production, which only occurs when an egg is released. Because estrogen secretion is unopposed, the uterine lining thickens and heavy uterine bleeding can result, causing heavy and painful periods at times. When the ovaries stop producing estrogen, the uterine lining does not thicken and there is no period. This is menopause.

Although ovulation stops, the central region of the ovary continues to make two hormones: *androstenedione* and *testosterone*. The adrenal glands, located on top of the kidneys, also produce androstenedione and testosterone, as well as small amounts of progesterone and estrogen. The liver, kidney, adrenals, brain, and fat cells take up the circulating androstenedione and convert it to estrogen and testosterone.

A steady supply of estrogen from your adrenal glands can help ease your transition through menopause. A healthy diet and exercise will help. It is important to maintain an adequate body weight (15 to 25 percent fat) so that there are enough fat cells to convert androstenedione into estrogen.

Figure 2.1
The Reproductive Cycle of Women: The Changes in Hormones, Ovarian Tissue, and Endometrium

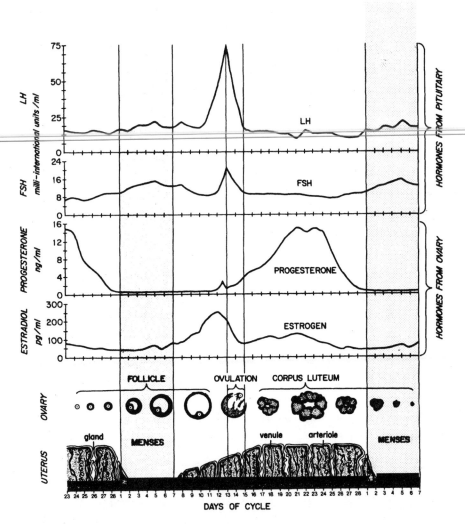

When Does Menopause Occur?

The average age of menopause is 51.2 years. That means half of all women will stop menstruating before they are this age and half of them will stop menstruating afterwards. Approximately 8 percent of women will experience menopause before the age of forty, and almost all will have experienced it by the age of fifty-eight.

Table 2.1 shows several factors, including smoking, that may result in an earlier onset of menopause.

Table 2.1
Causes of Premature or Early Menopause
(Less than 40 years old)

- Surgical removal of the ovaries
- Radiation therapy to the ovaries
- Mumps
- Chromosome deletion
- Severe malnutrition
- Autoimmune disease
- Smoking

Younger women can go through menopause as well. The most common cause of early menopause is the surgical removal of the ovaries. Ovaries are removed because of tumors, cancer, or pelvic inflammatory disease. However, both ovaries must be removed for menopause to occur. Even if a portion of one ovary is present, it can continue to produce eggs and hormones.

Women can also have a late menopause, that is, after the age of fifty-five. If you continue to menstruate well into your fifties, make sure that you have an annual Pap test, pelvic exam, and mammogram, and take extra care to do monthly breast self-exams (see appendix B). Your doctor should also know that you are continuing to menstruate, because at times vaginal bleeding may be abnormal.

Is There Any Test to Determine Whether You Are Menopausal?

Hot flashes and irregular cycles do not always mean that menopause is imminent. Obtaining an FSH level is the most useful test to determine whether you are in menopause. Because the ovary fails to produce estrogen, the FSH level rises as the pituitary attempts to make the ovaries produce more estrogen. Consequently, a high FSH level is a good indicator that you are menopausal. Your physician will be able to tell you whether you are perimenopausal or menopausal by the results of this test.

Summary

- Menopause occurs as the ovaries run out of eggs. Estrogen production falls and menstrual periods become irregular.

- The average age of menopause is 51.2 years.

- Early menopause can occur due to surgical removal of or radiation to the ovaries or chromosomal abnormalities.

- Some women menstruate well into their fifties. This is a normal variant. However, if you are in your fifties and are still menstruating, your risk for breast and uterine cancer increases. It is important to notify your physician and get a comprehensive annual physical exam.

- Measuring FSH level is the most useful way to determine whether you are menopausal.

3

Short-Term Effects of Menopause

There are a number of changes that you may experience as a result of menopause. Some of them begin during perimenopause, while others occur later and are the result of being without estrogen for a longer period of time. This chapter focuses on the short-term effects and will cover

- Changes in the menstrual cycle

- Hot flashes

- Mood changes

- Changes in the vagina

- Other changes associated with menopause

What Are the Changes Associated with Menopause?

Changes in Your Menstrual Cycle

Approximately 80 percent of all women will experience some kind of change in their cycle about seven years prior to menopause, with cycles becoming either more frequent or infrequent and periods becoming shorter or longer. These differences reflect the changes in hormonal production by your ovaries. If no follicles develop within the ovary, no estrogen is produced, and you will miss a cycle. If ovulation does not occur, estrogen production continues with a resultant thickening of the uterine lining, and when the lining sloughs off, heavy bleeding results. Alternatively, your cycle may be shorter because estrogen is not being

Table 3.1
What It Means

Symptom	Reason
Short cycles	Preovulatory estrogen is not being made. The follicular phase of your cycle will be less than 14 days. You still ovulate and have your period 2 weeks later, but your cycle is shorter.
Light bleeding	You are not producing as much estrogen. Your uterine lining will be thinner. When menstruation occurs, there will be less flow.
Heavy bleeding	You are not ovulating. Estrogen continues to stimulate the growth of the uterine lining with no progesterone to oppose it. Your lining will be thicker than usual, so when it is shed, blood flow will be heavier.
Missed period	No follicle develops so no estrogen is produced. The uterine lining does not thicken and is not sloughed off.

made in the preovulatory phase, so the follicular phase of your cycle is shorter and your period comes prematurely.

You may find it helpful to keep track of your menstrual periods as you approach menopause. This will allow you to record any irregularities in your period and highlight potential problems. The simplest thing to do is get a calendar and mark the day your period begins and ends. Note whether bleeding was light, moderate, or heavy. Note any other symptoms if appropriate; for example, cramps, breast soreness, bloating, or moodiness. If you have had spotting at another time of the month, note this and indicate the type of flow. If possible, estimate when ovulation occurred.

A calendar has been provided here for you to track your periods. First, a sample is given, followed by a blank calendar, which can be photocopied.

When to see your doctor

The following is a list of potential danger signs. While heavy bleeding or irregular cycles are frequently normal during the perimenopause, you should check with your physician if you have any of the following symptoms:

Sample Menstrual Cycle Calendar

Month _February, 1996_

SUN	MON	TUE	WED	THUR	FRI	SAT
				1	2	3
4	5	6	7	8	9	10
11	12	13	14	15	16 M	17 M
18 M	19 B=L	20 B=H C	21 B=M	22 B=L	23 B=L	24
25	26	27	28	29		

Directions:

1. Mark each day of your period by placing a diagonal line across the box.

2. For each day of your period, record your level of bleeding.

> "B=L" indicates light bleeding

> "B=M" indicates moderate bleeding

> "B=H" indicates heavy bleeding

3. If there were any days during which you had spotting, record an "S."

4. If you can estimate when ovulation occurred, mark that date with an "O."

5. If there were any days during which you experienced moodiness or mood swings, record an "M."

6. Create other symbols for your own use:

> _C_ = _Cramps_

> __ = _____

Menstrual Cycle Calendar

Month _____

SUN	MON	TUE	WED	THUR	FRI	SAT

- Extremely heavy, frequent, prolonged bleeding
- Bleeding between periods
- Bleeding during intercourse
- Bleeding that begins after you have not menstruated for about one year. **This is extremely important because it may be an early sign of cancer.**

Heavy periods

While some amount of heavy bleeding is common in the perimenopausal years, heavy blood flow can cause an iron-deficiency anemia with symptoms of fatigue, dizziness, and weakness. If you have heavy bleeding, you may want to supplement your diet with iron. However, there are other causes of anemia, including colon cancer and ulcers, so you should discuss this first with your physician. Chapter 4 discusses other conditions that can lead to heavy bleeding.

Tips for managing heavy bleeding. A few lifestyle changes can be helpful in managing heavy bleeding (See table 3.2). Factors that cause heavy bleeding include alcohol, aspirin, and heat.

Irregular bleeding

Irregular bleeding, even if slight, can also be a symptom of a serious health problem, such as cervical or uterine cancer. For this reason, you should note this on your menstrual calendar and report any irregular spotting or bleeding to your physician immediately.

Table 3.2
How to Minimize Heavy Bleeding

Avoid	Do
Alcohol—Heavy drinking affects the formation of blood platelets, which help the blood clot. With fewer platelets, blood will not clot as well.	Exercise—Regular aerobic exercise lowers the body's production of FSH and LH, which lowers estrogen production by the ovaries.
Aspirin*—Aspirin also increases bleeding by lowering the ability of platelets to clot.	Have your blood checked for signs of anemia.
Hot showers or baths—By dilating blood vessels, bleeding is increased.	

* Unless otherwise directed by your physician

Skipped periods

As you approach menopause, there may be some months in which you are not ovulating, and your uterus will not shed its lining. A missed period is often a cause of concern for women who may mistake it for a sign of pregnancy. If a missed period is accompanied by hot flashes and dryness in the vagina, it is more likely a sign of menopause. However, do not make any assumptions about pregnancy until you have further tests done at your doctor's office. Home pregnancy tests are not as reliable at this time in life and may be falsely positive.

Premenstrual syndrome

PMS starting in your late thirties can be an early indicator of perimenopause. It is characterized by monthly breast tenderness, bloating, weight gain, depression, anxiety, irritability, and insomnia.

Hot Flashes

The hot flash, the most common menopausal sign, is an episode of intense warmth in the upper body or a drenching sweat followed by chills. It may be preceded by a sense of anxiety, tension, dizziness, nausea, tingling in the fingers, and palpitations. Sometimes, it can manifest itself as a vague sense of "not feeling right."

Eighty percent of menopausal women have hot flashes. Frequency and individual experiences vary considerably. Hot flashes usually stop one to two years after the last period but may continue for up to ten years past that point. They may last from a few seconds to a few minutes, and tend to occur more frequently during the night. For most women, hot flashes are uncomfortable but bearable. For 10 to 15 percent, however, they can be quite debilitating.

What causes hot flashes?

During a hot flash, epinephrine (adrenaline) levels rise. It is unclear why this happens, but scientists believe that it may be caused by changes in the hypothalamus, which regulates body temperature along with the menstrual cycle. As a result, heart rate rises, and there is an increase in blood flow and body temperature.

The changes in the hypothalamus are brought about by declining estrogen levels. The more abrupt the drop in your estrogen level, the more severe your hot flashes. Further, thin women often have a more difficult time with hot flashes than heavy women. Researchers believe that heavier women continue to produce estrogen in their fat cells and thus have a more gradual decline in estrogen during menopause.

Managing your hot flashes

Keep track of when, under what circumstances (stress, certain foods), and how often your hot flashes occur. Often, it will become evident that there is a pattern. The following

---

Tips for Managing Your Hot Flashes

- *Watch your diet.* Try to avoid alcohol, caffeine, and spicy foods. Too much sugar, hot soups or drinks, and very large meals can also set off hot flashes.

- *Stop smoking.* Nicotine is known to increase and intensify hot flashes.

- *Keep cool.* Wear natural fibers that "breathe." At night, sleep with a sheet or light covers. Keep room temperatures at a comfortable level. Drink cool drinks and take cold showers. Cooling yourself with a fan or splashing your face with water can help.

- *Exercise.* Being physically active can decrease the severity of hot flashes. Exercise improves circulation and makes your body better able to tolerate temperature extremes and cool down quickly. It also increases the amount of estrogen and other hormones that are circulating, which will diminish the severity of the hot flash.

- *Reduce your stress level.* Stress can make hot flashes worse (see chapter 12).

- *Get medical help.* Replacing the estrogen that is lost during menopause is the most effective way of eliminating hot flashes. Because of potential side effects of estrogen use, however, this decision should be made carefully. For a more detailed discussion of hormone replacement therapy, see chapter 6.

---

chart will help you keep track of your hot flashes. This information can be useful in helping you to manage them. A sample has been provided first, in which hot flashes for one day have been recorded. This is followed by a blank chart, which you are encouraged to photocopy.

Sleep Changes

Women can experience restless, fragmented sleep five to seven years before menopause. Changes in your sleeping patterns may be the earliest indicators of hormonal change. Sleep loss affects people in different ways and can lead to problems such as lack of concentration, memory loss, irritability, fatigue, and muscle aches and pains.

Mood Changes

Recent studies suggest that estrogen enhances mood in healthy, nondepressed adult women, even before menopause. In addition, changes in mood are often reported as women reach menopause and estrogen levels drop. Besides the decrease in estrogen, there may be other possible causes for the mood changes. If you have already been diagnosed as having PMS, clinical depression, or have ongoing emotional problems, you may find that your

Sample Hot Flash Chart

From: 2/4   **To:** 2/10

	SUNDAY	MONDAY	TUESDAY	WEDNESDAY	THURSDAY	FRIDAY	SATURDAY
#1	T: 1:30 A.M. Intensity: 7 Possible Causes: N	T: Intensity: Possible Causes:	T: Intensity: Possible Causes:	T: Intensity: Possible Causes:	T: Intensity: Possible Causes:	T: Intensity: Possible Causes:	T: Intensity: Possible Causes:
#2	T: 8:00 A.M. Intensity: 6 Possible Causes: **Ex, Cof**	T: Intensity: Possible Causes:	T: Intensity: Possible Causes:	T: Intensity: Possible Causes:	T: Intensity: Possible Causes:	T: Intensity: Possible Causes:	T: Intensity: Possible Causes:
#3	T: 12:30 P.M. Intensity: 6 Possible Causes: **Cof, St**	T: Intensity: Possible Causes:	T: Intensity: Possible Causes:	T: Intensity: Possible Causes:	T: Intensity: Possible Causes:	T: Intensity: Possible Causes:	T: Intensity: Possible Causes:
#4	T: 11:30 P.M. Intensity: 7 Possible Causes: N	T: Intensity: Possible Causes:	T: Intensity: Possible Causes:	T: Intensity: Possible Causes:	T: Intensity: Possible Causes:	T: Intensity: Possible Causes:	T: Intensity: Possible Causes:

Directions:

1. Record the time of your hot flash.
2. Rate its intensity from 1–10, with higher numbers indicating greater severity.
3. Note any possible causes—anything you did or experienced that could have precipitated the flash. Choose from the following list, using the highlighted letters in each word as a code:

Alcohol	**C**igarette	**C**offee	**E**xercise	**H**eavy Clothing	**H**ot **F**ood
Forgot **HRT**	**N**ight	**St**ress	**Sp**icy **F**ood	**W**arm **E**nvironment

Others (add your own): _____

Hot Flash Chart

Month/Week From: _____ **To:** _____

	SUNDAY	MONDAY	TUESDAY	WEDNESDAY	THURSDAY	FRIDAY	SATURDAY
#1	T: Intensity: Possible Causes:	T: Intensity: Possible Causes:	T: Intensity: Possible Causes:	T: Intensity: Possible Causes:	T: Intensity: Possible Causes:	T: Intensity: Possible Causes:	T: Intensity: Possible Causes:
#2	T: Intensity: Possible Causes:	T: Intensity: Possible Causes:	T: Intensity: Possible Causes:	T: Intensity: Possible Causes:	T: Intensity: Possible Causes:	T: Intensity: Possible Causes:	T: Intensity: Possible Causes:
#3	T: Intensity: Possible Causes:	T: Intensity: Possible Causes:	T: Intensity: Possible Causes:	T: Intensity: Possible Causes:	T: Intensity: Possible Causes:	T: Intensity: Possible Causes:	T: Intensity: Possible Causes:
#4	T: Intensity: Possible Causes:	T: Intensity: Possible Causes:	T: Intensity: Possible Causes:	T: Intensity: Possible Causes:	T: Intensity: Possible Causes:	T: Intensity: Possible Causes:	T: Intensity: Possible Causes:

Directions:

1. Record the time of your hot flash.
2. Rate its intensity from 1–10, with higher numbers indicating greater severity.
3. Note any possible causes—anything you did or experienced that could have precipitated the flash. Choose from the following list, using the highlighted letters in each word as a code:

Alcohol   **C**igarette   **C**offee   **E**xercise   **H**eavy Clothing   **H**ot Food

Forgot **HRT**   **N**ight   **S**tress   **S**picy Food   **W**arm Environment

Others (add your own): _____

4. If you wish to record more than four hot flashes per day, simply photocopy this chart.

Tips for Dealing with Sleep Deprivation

- Maintain a regular schedule. Wake up and go to sleep at around the same time each day.

- Avoid caffeine and alcohol, which affect sleep.

- Avoid over-the-counter drugs such as nasal decongestants, antihistamines, and diet aids, which can affect sleep.

- Stop smoking. Nicotine acts as a stimulant.

- Exercise on a regular basis. However, do not exercise too close to bedtime, as it can be overly stimulating.

- Take a hot bath before you go to bed. Raising your body temperature is a way to induce deeper, longer lasting sleep. However, hot baths may also trigger hot flashes in some women.

- Drink milk at bedtime.

- Adjust the temperature of your bedroom.

- Sleep in light cotton clothing with a minimal amount of bedding. Avoid polyester and nylon, either in nightclothes or sheets, as they hold the perspiration next to your body and can intensify your discomfort.

---

symptoms become exacerbated during perimenopause. For more information about mood changes, see chapter 10.

Changes in the Vagina and Urethra

As your estrogen level drops, the tissues of the vagina and urethra become thinner and drier. Sexual intercourse may become painful and uncomfortable and sexual arousal can take longer with less lubrication. Vaginal infections and a decrease or loss of sexual drive may occur.

Other Short-Term Effects

There are other miscellaneous changes that can occur with low estrogen levels that are generally less frequent and less severe than those mentioned above. These changes include crawling skin (formication), headaches, memory loss, and fatigue. They only affect a small percentage of women, are temporary, and disappear after menopause.

Tips for Dealing with Vaginal Dryness

- Regular sex is one of the best cures for vaginal dryness. This entails achieving orgasm once or twice a week with a partner or by masturbation. Sex increases the blood flow to your vagina, stimulates the mucous membrane, and exercises the surrounding tissue.

- Use lubricants. There are several over-the-counter lubricants such as Astroglide, K-Y Jelly, or Replens. You can also have your physician prescribe estrogen cream.

- Wear the right underclothes. Vaginal dryness can lead to itching and the growth of bacteria, which can lead to infection. Wear panties and panty hose with cotton crotches to allow the air to circulate.

Crawling Skin (Formication)

This symptom can occur during perimenopause. It feels like an itchy, crawling sensation and will respond to estrogen. It usually disappears during menopause.

Headaches

After menopause, some women with menstrual migraines will stop having headaches while others will report an increase in the frequency of their headaches. You can keep a record of your headaches on your hot flash chart. Identify any potential triggers including food, alcohol, stress levels, and amount of sleep. By doing this, you may be able to identify what sets off your headaches.

In addition to cutting out triggers, it is helpful to know that exercise and sexual activity diminish migraines. If you are on hormone replacement therapy (HRT) and you are having headaches, you might want to try a different brand of hormones.

Memory Loss

It is not uncommon for women to experience short-term memory loss around the time of perimenopause. This appears to be temporary and is helped by HRT. It is probably related to lack of sleep, stress, or the normal aging process.

Whenever anyone experiences memory problems it is quite disconcerting, and many people will become concerned about Alzheimer's disease or related problems. It helps to know that age does not affect intelligence. If you were smart when you were younger, you will maintain this into old age. Older people remember almost as much as younger people, with the main difference being that it often takes them longer to retrieve the information. Only 5 to 7 percent of women show serious intellectual impairment after the age of sixty-five.

Tips for Dealing with Memory Loss

- Use notes, lists, and day planners.

- Use bright color-coded tabs and highlighters. Bright colors grab your attention and are remembered more easily (for example, use purple ink on green notepaper).

- Use or create acronyms by combining the first letters of key words to be remembered. For example, an acronym for the names of the Great Lakes would be HOMES—Huron, Ontario, Michigan, Erie, Superior.

- Create a mnemonic device by using the first letter of each word to be remembered to make a sentence or rhyme. For example, a common mnemonic for the lines in the treble clef music staff of E, G, B, D, F, is "Every Good Boy Does Fine."

- Associate information to be remembered with knowledge and life experiences you already have. For example, associate a phone number with someone's birthday or anniversary (228-1954 could be your son's birthday on 2/28/54).

- Use input from a variety of senses to reinforce learning. For example, read the information to be remembered, write it down, and repeat it out loud.

- Create mental images or a series of pictures for the information to be remembered. The pictures should be absurd or unusual to enhance recall. For example, to remember Dr. Steinman's name, associate it with a man holding an enormous beer stein).

- Rehearse (recite/repeat) the material to be remembered.

- Review new information immediately, since research suggests that most forgetting occurs in the first few minutes after the information is taken in. For example, as soon as someone is introduced to you, use their name in your next sentence.

If memory loss persists after menopause or is disabling, you should seek medical advice. High blood pressure, some medications, vitamin deficiencies, anemia, sleep loss, or stress can affect memory.

How Serious Are Your Menopausal Changes?

By completing the following chart, you will find out to what degree you suffer from menopausal changes.

Table 3.3
Menopausal Distress Severity

0 = None	1 = Mild	2 = Moderate	3 = Severe

Symptom	Severity (0–3)
Hot flashen/Night sweats	
Vaginal dryness	
Prickling/burning	
Insomnia	
Mood changes/depression	
Nervousness	
Weakness (fatigue)	
Headaches	
Memory loss	
Formication (itchy feeling on skin)	
Other:	
	Total:

0–8 = Mild

8–20 = Moderate

21+ = Severe

Summary

A general knowledge of what is happening in your body can help to reassure you that menopause is natural and normal. It is also important to be aware of changes in your menstrual cycle so you can consult with your health care provider. In most cases, medical intervention will not be necessary.

Here is a list of possible short-term menopausal changes:

- Changes in the menstrual cycle

- PMS

- Hot flashes

- Sleep changes

- Mood changes
- Vaginal dryness
- Changes in sex drive

Less common changes include:

- Crawling skin
- Headaches
- Memory loss
- Heart palpitations
- Fatigue

4

Long-Term Effects of Menopause

Like the short-term effects, the long-term physical effects of menopause are also due to decreased estrogen production. Some of these physical effects can be very serious, including

- Coronary heart disease (CHD)

- Osteoporosis

- Genitourinary problems, especially Stress Urinary Incontinence

In addition, there are more minor, cosmetic problems associated with menopause, such as skin, breast, and hair changes. This chapter will discuss these long-term changes and provide suggestions about how to manage them.

Coronary Heart Disease

Coronary heart disease (CHD) is one of the most serious developments that can occur after menopause. Unusual in women before menopause, CHD is a leading cause of death in women after menopause, exceeding that of all cancers. A fifty-year-old woman has a one in two chance of developing coronary heart disease in her lifetime. Almost one in three women will die from it.

Coronary heart disease develops when there is narrowing of one or more of the blood vessels carrying blood to the heart. As you age, there is a slow accumulation of cholesterol material within the walls of the blood vessels that supply the heart. These vessels become narrower as the cholesterol plaque continues to grow (see sketch 1). Consequently, there is

Blood Vessels Carrying Blood to the Heart

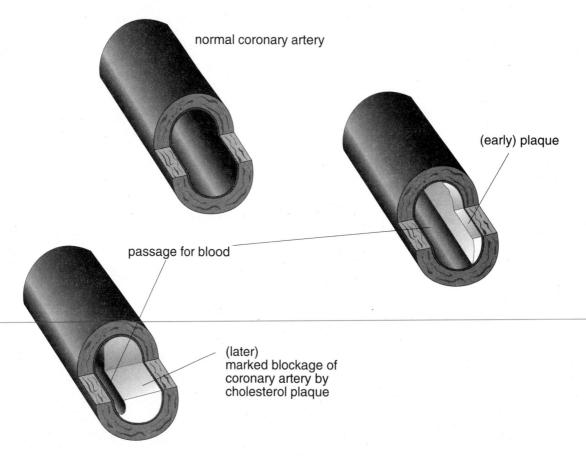

normal coronary artery

(early) plaque

passage for blood

(later)
marked blockage of
coronary artery by
cholesterol plaque

a decrease in blood flow to the heart muscle itself. The heart cannot pump the blood in a normal fashion and is therefore more prone to irregular heartbeats (*arrhythmias*).

As the blood flow to the heart decreases, and under physical exertion, women (and men) can experience a particular type of chest pain called *angina pectoris*. This is a crushing midchest pain that can radiate to the left arm or neck. Prolonged episodes of angina pectoris can cause some of the heart muscle to die. This is called a *heart attack*, or a *myocardial infarction*. As the heart muscle continues to deteriorate, the heart can no longer pump blood efficiently, and blood pools in the lungs. When this happens, it is called *congestive heart failure*. CHD is still considered to be a disease generally afflicting men. Reflecting the gender bias of most health studies, much of the research on heart disease has been done only on men. Often, however, women will not have classic symptoms and their heart attacks may go unnoticed. Women's symptoms may include being nauseated, tired, or just not feeling well. Women tend to develop coronary heart disease some ten years later than men and have their first heart attack in their sixties, some years after menopause. They also tend to die at a higher rate from the initial heart attack than men, because their heart attacks occur later and their symptoms can be atypical and thus misdiagnosed.

What protects the premenopausal woman's heart?

It is thought that the major protective factor is estrogen. The presence of estrogen reduces the circulating low-density lipoprotein (LDL), or "bad cholesterol," and increases the high-density lipoprotein (HDL), or "good cholesterol." HDL removes cholesterol from the bloodstream, whereas LDL brings cholesterol into the blood stream. Researchers also feel that estrogen may decrease the formation of blood clots within these arteries. In addition, estrogen tends to dilate, or widen, coronary arteries, allowing more blood flow to the heart.

As you go through menopause, there is a gradual decline in the level of circulating estrogen, which means you will lose its protection in preventing the development of heart disease.

Biological risk factors

Some women are at greater risk of developing heart disease than others. The following table lists the biological risk factors for the development of coronary heart disease:

Table 4.1
Biological Risk Factors for Coronary Heart Disease (CHD)

Check all risk factors that apply to you. Discuss any "yes" or "don't know" answers with your physician and develop a plan to minimize or treat the conditions.

	Yes	No	Don't Know
Cigarette smoking			
High blood pressure			
Diabetes			
Obesity			
Oophorectomy			
Postmenopausal and not using HRT			
Family history of first heart attack before age 60			
Elevated cholesterol			
Elevated triglycerides			
Advanced age (71 to 80)			
African-American			

Psychological risk factors

There continues to be controversy as to whether the type-A personality (the compulsively driven, competitive workaholic) contributes to the development of coronary heart disease. Studies trying to determine whether there is a relationship between type-A personality and the development of heart disease are not conclusive, partly because they were done on white males only.

Prevention of heart disease

On a positive note, you can reduce your chances of developing heart disease by reducing the risk factors you have. All of the following can help:

- Eliminating cigarette smoking

- Aggressively treating high blood pressure, if it exists

- Controlling diabetes

- Maintaining a normal body weight for your age and height

- Treating elevated cholesterol and triglyceride levels through diet, exercise, and, if indicated, medication

- Using hormone replacement therapy (this can reduce heart disease by 50 percent)

In addition, there are other things that you can do to prevent or slow down the development of heart disease. Among these are good nutrition and exercise, which are discussed in chapter 8.

While the treatment of coronary heart disease is beyond the scope of this book, if you do have it, it is important to have a good collaborative relationship with your physician or health care provider. This will help in the prevention and treatment of further cardiac problems. See chapter 15 for advice on establishing this relationship.

Osteoporosis

Osteoporosis, or "porous bones," is another of the most serious health problems related to menopause. Bone is constantly being broken down and replaced. Osteoporosis occurs when more bone is broken down than is built, causing bone loss to occur. Bones then break more easily, resulting in broken hips and wrists, and compression fractures of the vertebra (which are responsible for the loss of height and curvature of the spine). Estrogen protects bones from calcium loss. However, at menopause, when the levels of estrogen are dropping, there is a loss of bone density. This loss occurs most rapidly in the first five years of menopause, when bone loss can reach 3 to 4 percent of the total bone mass.

About one out of every three postmenopausal women has, or is in the process of developing, osteoporosis. Over a million women will develop fractures due to osteoporosis, and 25 to 30 percent of these will be hip fractures. The total medical cost of treating this disorder and its complications is around $10 billion per year. That does not take into account the human toll in pain and suffering. In 25 percent of Caucasian and Asian women, compression fractures of the vertebra and wrists begin at age sixty. Consequently, these women will become shorter and, as they age, will develop the classic "dowager's hump."

Fractures can have serious consequences. Around 20 percent of women undergoing hip replacement surgery after a hip fracture will die within one year of their injuries, a death rate that is greater than that of cancer of the breast and uterus combined. (The death is usually due to blood and fat clots released from the fracture site.) Approximately half of these women will require constant nursing care as a result of the hip fracture.

The main risk for developing osteoporosis is related to bone mass. If you have more bone mass, your chances of developing osteoporosis are reduced. Table 4.2 lists some other risk factors.

Evaluation of osteoporosis

Osteoporosis is usually asymptomatic and not recognized until a fracture occurs. At least 25 percent of bone has to be lost before osteoporosis can be diagnosed from a routine X ray. There are a variety of tests other than routine X rays for measuring bone mineral content. DEXA (Duo Energy X-ray Absorptiometry) is currently felt to be the best test available. It is a painless procedure that scans an image of your hip and spine. A computer compares your bone density with the bone density of a young adult and of someone your age. Once performed only at major medical centers, bone density tests are now widely available. Many doctors will recommend this test if you have a number of the risk factors for osteoporosis. Make sure you go to a facility that has a lot of experience in performing these tests. Biochemical markers, such as Osteomark, are now being used to test for bone turnover.

Prevention of osteoporosis

Getting an adequate amount of calcium as an adolescent is one of the most important factors in preventing osteoporosis because it is in adolescence that the greatest amount of bone mass is laid down. However, most studies show that adolescent girls get far less than their minimum daily requirement (800–1200 mg) of calcium per day, placing them at risk for the development of osteoporosis.

Exercise may also play a part in the prevention of osteoporosis. This is especially true if you have been sedentary. However, no one has quantified the intensity of exercise required to have a positive effect on the skeletal system. While exercise can increase bone density, it will not, by itself, prevent osteoporosis. The beneficial effects of exercise will last only as long as it is continued.

Many studies have shown that hormone replacement therapy reduces the amount of postmenopausal bone loss, as well as the incidence of fractures, and is considered to be the best prevention for osteoporosis. Five years of estrogen therapy will reduce the risk of developing fractures by half. The minimum daily dosage of estrogen needed to prevent osteoporosis is 0.625 mg of Premarin, 0.625 mg of estrone sulfate, or .5 mg of estradiol. Transdermal patches may also decrease the loss of bone mass. Chapter 6 will explain more about HRT and help you make the decision that's right for you.

Table 4.2
Risk Factors for Osteoporosis

Check all risk factors that apply to you. Discuss any "yes" answers with your physician and develop a plan to minimize or treat.

	Yes	No
Caucasian or Asian		
Very thin		
Early menopause (before age 40)		
Surgical menopause		
Family history of osteoporosis		
Low calcium intake (<1500 mg/day)		
Low vitamin D intake		
High caffeine intake		
High alcohol intake		
High protein intake		
Cigarette smoking		
Sedentary lifestyle		
Endocrine disorder		
Diabetes		
Hyperthyroidism		
Cushing's disease		
Hyperparathyroidism		
Steroid therapy for more than 6 months		
Postmenopausal and not on HRT		

Table 4.3
A Prescription for the Prevention of Osteoporosis

- 1000 mg calcium per day for premenopausal women

- 1500 mg of calcium per day for postmenopausal women

- Exercise

- Decrease risk factors (see table 4.2)

- The use of HRT early in menopause (see chapter 6)

Treatment of osteoporosis

As mentioned earlier, exercise may also have a positive effect on bone mass. Remember, exercise is *only* an adjunct, *not* an alternative to estrogen replacement for the treatment of osteoporosis in menopausal women. For more about exercise, see chapter 8.

New treatments for osteoporosis

These medications help increase bone density and stop bone loss before fractures occur. They are intended for postmenopausal women who already have low bone density.

- *Fossamax* (alendronate) decreases bone loss and increases bone density. It is more potent than *Didronel* (etidronate), which is also used to treat osteoporosis. It also has fewer side effects, such as diarrhea and nausea. Fossamax is available by prescription.

- *Miacalcin* (calcitonin) has been released as a nasal spray. It decreases bone loss, like Fossamax and Didronel, but it doesn't increase bone density.

- *Slow release fluoride* stimulates new bone formation. If calcium citrate is added, stronger bone is produced. Slow release fluoride is not widely recommended because it is associated with a higher incidence of vertebral fractures and has not yet received FDA approval.

Genitourinary Systems

Some changes in the vagina and urethra have already been discussed in chapter 3. In addition to these, the vulva (the lips surrounding the vaginal opening) become thinner. The vulva may also shrink, making the vaginal opening too tight for comfortable sexual intercourse. When this happens, intercourse can cause pain and irritation of the urethra.

Bladder problems

Stress Urinary Incontinence (SUI) refers to the involuntary loss of urine when you laugh, cough, or sneeze. Stress Urinary Incontinence occurs because the urethra begins to stretch away from the pubic bone. This can occur prior to menopause, but is most disturbing after age sixty. Vaginal births and years of standing and straining can make this condition more likely.

Fifty percent of women with SUI can avoid surgery if they have good pelvic muscle tone and practice the Kegel exercise (see box below). If you do these exercises for approximately two minutes four times a day, it will take about two to three months before incontinence stops. If the exercises are discontinued, the incontinence will return. For the remaining women, collagen injections around the urethra can build support or surgery can be done. About 75 percent of women with SUI will no longer have symptoms after surgery.

The Kegel Exercise

Dr. Arnold Kegel invented this exercise in the 1950s. It helps to strengthen the pubococcygeal muscle, which helps you stop the flow of urine and prevent a bowel movement. It also is the muscle that contracts during orgasm.

1. Locate your pelvic floor muscles by pretending to stop the flow of urine while urinating. Alternatively, you can contract the anal sphincter as you would to prevent a bowel movement. You will feel a distinct tightening of your muscles.

2. Tighten these muscles again, hold for 10 seconds, and then release. Repeat this 10 times.

3. Repeat 5 to 10 times each day.

Since no one will be aware that you are doing this exercise, you can do it anywhere—while watching television, in the car at a stoplight, or at your desk during the day. The important thing is to make it a daily habit.

Skin Changes

Skin thickness declines at the same rate as bone density. Thirty percent of skin collagen (connective tissue) is lost in the first ten years after the onset of menopause. The skin bruises easily, and may have either increased pigmentation—called "liver spots"—or decreased pigmentation. Facial acne can also appear. The breasts can lose fatty tissue and elasticity, which leads to smaller, sagging breasts. Wrinkles, another common age-related skin change, are caused primarily by sun damage and years of facial expressions.

Tips to Minimize Wrinkles

- Wear sunscreen daily and minimize your exposure to the sun.

- There is some evidence that HRT can be helpful.

- Don't drink or smoke. Alcohol and smoking are both associated with an increase in wrinkles.

- Maintain a healthy diet and lifestyle including plenty of water, exercise, and adequate rest.

- Some antioxidant vitamins (A, C, and E) seem to benefit the skin.

- Retin-A is used by many dermatologists for wrinkles caused by sun damage and for brown "age" spots.

- Alpha-hydroxy acids, such as lactic acid and glycolic acid, can be purchased over the counter, frequently in moisturizers. They act in a manner similar to Retin-A, but with less effectiveness, as well as fewer side effects.

- Dermabrasion, chemical peels, laser techniques, and cosmetic surgery are more invasive ways of treating wrinkles.

Hair Changes

As a result of the hormonal changes of menopause and aging, you are likely to notice changes in your hair that may include

- Thinning of scalp and pubic hair

- Loss of luster

Complete baldness is unlikely, but if your hair loss persists, you may want to consult a dermatologist. There is no treatment to restore the luster of the hair, unless it is due to hairstyling products and techniques. Graying of hair is hereditary, and is not reversed by HRT.

Hirsutism is the growth of dark, thick hair on the chin, lip, or neck, or around the nipples due to excessive androgenic hormones. You will want to consult with your physician if it develops since there are other causes of hirsutism that should be evaluated. For benign excessive hair growth, treatment alternatives include HRT, shaving, tweezing, waxing, bleaching, electrolysis, and depilatories. If you use a depilatory, make sure it is specifically developed for facial use and that you are not allergic to it.

Summary

Heart disease, osteoporosis, some genitourinary problems, and changes in the skin and hair can occur as a result of menopause.

- Coronary heart disease is no longer viewed only as a male disease.

- The death rate following heart attacks is higher for women than for men.

- Prevention or early interventions, such as diet, exercise, and HRT can reduce the incidence, severity, and mortality of heart disease.

- Osteoporosis remains a costly illness in terms of complications and health care dollars. Adequate calcium intake and exercise throughout the adolescent and adult years can help prevent this disease.

- HRT, when initiated early in menopause, helps to prevent osteoporosis.

- For those who cannot or choose not to use HRT, there are alternatives to aid in the prevention of bone loss.

- Kegel exercise and HRT can treat Stress Urinary Incontinence.

5

Hysterectomy

This chapter will discuss

- The types of hysterectomy

- The reasons for hysterectomy

- Making the decision about hysterectomy

- Alternatives to hysterectomy

- The physical and psychological aftereffects

- How to cope with the aftereffects

Hysterectomy and Surgical Menopause

Hysterectomy is a surgical procedure in which the uterus is removed. It is the most common major surgical procedure performed on menopausal women, affecting over one third of American women. Many people have felt that the incidence of hysterectomy in the United States has been too high, and that economic and social forces have determined its use as much as standard medical practice. In recent years—owing to pressure from the women's movement, the presence of an increasing number of female physicians, the development of partnerships between physicians and patients rather than paternalism, and the intrusion of market forces (that is, managed care)—the number of hysterectomies in the United States has been declining.

In addition to the removal of the uterus, hysterectomy almost always includes removal of the cervix as well. When this is done, it is called a *total hysterectomy*. Removal of the tubes and ovaries is called a *bilateral salpingo-oophorectomy*. In menopausal women, bilateral salpingo-oophorectomy and total hysterectomy are often done together, since the ovaries are not producing significant amounts of estrogen and can be a site for the development of ovarian cancer.

Table 5.1
Terms for the Removal of:

	Uterus	Cervix	Tubes and Ovaries
Hysterectomy	X		
Total hysterectomy	X	X	
Bilateral salpingo-oophorectomy			X

The decision to have a hysterectomy should not be taken lightly, because the operation can have significant postoperative complications including bleeding or infection. The death rate in nonmenopausal women under the age of fifty-four without cancer is six per ten thousand women. In addition, as women age, it takes longer to heal from surgical procedures.

Abnormal Uterine Bleeding and Alternatives to Hysterectomy

Of all hysterectomies done, almost one third are done because of fibroids and the resultant bleeding. However, not all abnormal uterine bleeding is caused by fibroids. Table 5.3 shows a list of causes of abnormal bleeding. If you are experiencing irregular bleeding, there are two evaluation procedures that you may want to discuss with your physician:

- *Ultrasound*, which can measure the lining of the uterus to determine if the bleeding is due to polyps, fibroids, or cancer. If the ultrasound is abnormal, your physician will likely do a *Dilatation and Curettage* (D & C), which can help with the diagnosis, and may also treat the problem.

Table 5.2
Reasons for Hysterectomy

Here are a handful of medical conditions for which hysterectomy is the best option:

- Invasive cervical, ovarian, or endometrial cancer
- Uncontrolled bleeding
- Severe pelvic infection which can't be controlled by antibiotics

Hysterectomy may often be done for other appropriate reasons, such as:

- Fibroids (muscular growths of the uterine wall)
- Abnormal bleeding
- Extensive endometriosis (the existence of endometrial tissue outside of the uterus)
- Precancerous conditions of the reproductive organs
- Prolapse of the uterus
- Chronic pelvic pain
- Recurrent pelvic infections

Table 5.3
Causes of Abnormal Vaginal and Uterine Bleeding

- Vaginitis (vaginal infections or inflammation)
- Cervicitis (inflammation of the cervix)
- Cervical or endometrial polyps (noncancerous growths of the cervix or lining of the uterus)
- Fibroids
- Clotting defects
- Medical disorders such as thyroid problems
- Medications, such as some antidepressants and hormones

Serious Causes of Abnormal Uterine Bleeding

- Endometrial hyperplasia (precancerous changes of the uterine lining)
- Cancer of the cervix, uterus, ovaries, or tubes

- *Hysteroscopy*, in which a fiber-optic instrument is inserted into the uterus. The hysteroscope is able to biopsy uterine tissue.

Depending upon the problem, there are a number of alternative treatments to hysterectomy. See table 5.4.

If fibroids are the source of bleeding, a class of medications called *gonadotropin releasing hormones* (GNRH), including Synarel and Lupron, can be used to help shrink the size of the fibroids. However, 60 percent of the fibroids return to the same size in six months. A hysterectomy or myomectomy should be done only when there are significant symptoms from the fibroid, such as painful pressure on the bladder or rectum, and when other treatments, such as D & Cs and hormones have failed to resolve the problem. Rapidly growing fibroids may require surgery.

Another possible treatment for abnormal bleeding, in the absence of cancer, is a procedure called *endometrial ablation*. In this treatment, an electrical current or a laser beam is applied to the lining of the uterus to stop the bleeding.

Making the Decision for Hysterectomy

If surgery is recommended for your bleeding, do not feel pressured into doing it. Before agreeing, you should always get a second opinion. Questions you should ask your physician include

- Can we give it more time to see if the problem clears up on its own?

- What will happen if I choose to do nothing?

- Can the problem be managed with medication?

- Are there any alternatives to surgery?

If you need a hysterectomy, it is important to find a gynecologist who is experienced in doing the procedure. You should ask

- Is it a vaginal or abdominal hysterectomy?

- How long will the procedure take?

- How long will I be in the hospital?

- What kind of anesthesia will be used?

- What are the possible complications?

- How much will it cost and does that include the follow-up care?

- How long will it take to recover, and what will the recovery period be like?

- When can I start having sex again?

Table 5.4
Alternatives to Hysterectomy

Conditions	Alternatives
Fibroids	Myomectomy (removal of the fibroid)
	Lupron
	Synarel
Endometriosis	Danazol
	Lupron
	Synarel
Precancerous conditions	D & C
	Cervical conization
	Hormonal treatment
Uterine prolapse	Estrogen cream
	Pessary
Abnormal (noncancerous) uterine bleeding	Progesterone
	Birth control pills
	Estrogen
	Endometrial ablation
Pelvic pain	Psychological evaluation and treatment, if appropriate
	Nonsteroidal anti-inflammatory drugs
	Pain management

The Aftereffects of Hysterectomy

Physical Aftereffects

Removing both the uterus and ovaries can cause the immediate onset of menopause, which can be devastating. Unless a woman starts immediately on hormone replacement therapy and stays on it, she can have all of the physical changes associated with menopause. There will also be an increased risk of the premature onset of osteoporosis, as well as of heart disease.

One in seventy women will develop ovarian cancer. Because it is very difficult to detect, it has an extremely high mortality rate. Ovarian cancer causes more deaths than any cancer of the female reproductive tract. This is one of the reasons many physicians prefer to remove the ovaries at the time of hysterectomy in menopausal women. Presently, there is a blood test called *CA-125*, which, along with the use of ultrasound, can be used to monitor the presence or absence of cancer in the ovaries. However, the CA-125 has a high degree (15 to 40 percent) of false positives—this means that a lot of women who have a positive test result may not have cancer. The use of these screening tests (CA-125 and ultrasound) may prevent the necessity of oophorectomy.

Some 10 to 40 percent of women complain of sexual dysfunction after hysterectomy. The most common problems are painful intercourse, decreased orgasm due to an absence of uterine contractions, and decreased sexual desire. Women whose ovaries were removed at the time of hysterectomy are most likely to have sexual complaints. Women may also experience a reduction in sexual functioning if there is a prior history of depression, sexual difficulties, or other psychological difficulties. The women who seem to do best in terms of their sexual functioning and express satisfaction after hysterectomy are the ones who had clear-cut reasons for hysterectomy, severe medical problems, understood and consented to the surgery, and had active and satisfactory sex lives before surgery.

Psychological Aftereffects

The uterus is important to women for many reasons. Even if a woman does not want children or has had children and does not want any more, a hysterectomy can be a loss. Having a hysterectomy is often seen as a threat to health, femininity, identity, or sexuality.

Some researchers believe that serious depression can occur in women who have lost the ability to bear children before they've had a chance to conceive. These researchers suggest that within two to three years of surgery, a significant percentage of women will experience an episode of depression. Women who have a greater risk for becoming clinically depressed have had a history of a prior depressive episode, anxiety, sexual difficulties, or have had the hysterectomy performed for unclear reasons. However, other researchers found no evidence that hysterectomy is followed by a higher rate of depression. Future careful research will be needed to clarify this apparent contradiction.

If you are going to have a hysterectomy with an oophorectomy, here are some suggestions to optimize the outcome:

- You may want to consider hormone replacement therapy.

- You will need yearly Pap smears, since cancer can still develop in the vaginal vault.

- You will be less likely to become depressed if you understand what will be happening to your body after the surgery and why you are having the surgery.

- You will also do better if you have the support of your partner and have ample social support.

- You may have a period of time during which psychological issues will arise.

- Allow yourself time to recover, to mourn your losses, and to deal with the psychological issues as they arise.

Summary

- Hysterectomy at times can be lifesaving and can significantly improve your health.

- Unnecessary hysterectomy can have disabling consequences.

- There are alternatives to hysterectomy and these should be discussed with your health care provider.

- If you are a premenopausal woman, removal of the uterus and ovaries can plunge you quickly into menopause, causing all of the changes that are seen in a normal menopause. Consequently, you are at risk for the development of heart disease, osteoporosis, and the other physical changes that are associated with menopause.

- Hormone replacement therapy should be considered if physical changes associated with menopause occur, and may prevent or slow some of the changes if it is instituted quickly enough.

- Pap smears are suggested yearly if you who have had a hysterectomy for cancer of the cervix. They should be done even though you have had a hysterectomy, since cancer can occur in the vaginal vault.

- An ongoing dialogue between you and your health care provider is required so that you will get optimal care.

6

Hormone Replacement Therapy

The development of hormone replacement therapy, or HRT—the use of estrogen and progesterone following the menopause—began in the 1940s. Few areas of women's health stir up as much controversy as HRT, because studies on the use of hormones are often conflicting, and most have their critics. To take or not take hormones will be one of the biggest medical decisions you will have to make.

This chapter will discuss

- The effects of HRT on changes associated with menopause

- The side effects of HRT

- The risks of HRT

- How to decide whether or not to use HRT

Presently, it is estimated that almost 20 percent (seven to eight million) of American women over the age of forty-five are on hormone replacement therapy. The average length of treatment is between nine and twelve months. A large percentage of these women do not refill their prescription after six months or less because they find that monthly bleeding is unacceptable or that the side effects of the hormones are debilitating. A small number quit because they no longer need the short-term physical or psychological benefits of hormones.

Table 6.1
HRT at a Glance

Hormone	What it does
Estrogen	This class of hormones stimulates the production of proteins that maintain the vagina, uterus, breast, and bone. It also helps regulate body temperature and influences cholesterol production. Hot flashes, vaginal dryness, bone loss, decreased breast tissue, and increased serum cholesterol are among some of the things that happen as the result of the reduction of estrogen after menopause.
Progestogen	Progestogen, a substance that mimics progesterone, prevents the abnormal growth of the uterine lining, a condition known as *endometrial hyperplasia*.
Testosterone	While this hormone does not drop as dramatically after menopause, lower levels are associated with thinning pubic hair, loss of energy, reduced muscle mass, and lower libido. Most women take testosterone to enhance their sex drive. Testosterone is effective only in women whose levels are below the normal range (20–60 nanograms/dl).

What Does Hormone Replacement Therapy Do?

Hot Flashes

HRT will relieve some changes associated with menopause. Because low estrogen level is the cause of hot flashes, estrogen treatment almost always relieves them. Studies show that other medications, such as sedatives, Clonidine (an antihypertensive drug), vitamin E, and placebos are not as effective as HRT. Exercise also does not alleviate hot flashes, although it may make them more tolerable. With time, the hot flashes will diminish, although they may continue in some women for ten years or more after menopause. You should know that if you are on HRT and go off of it, hot flashes may return.

Vaginal Changes

The lack of estrogen can also produce vaginal dryness and with it, painful intercourse. Taking estrogen will solve this problem. However, you will need to continue to take estrogen to maintain this effect. Estrogen will also help the vagina retain its acidity, which makes it more resistant to infections.

Stress Urinary Incontinence and Urinary Tract Infections

Some gynecologists feel that pelvic tone will not be strengthened by estrogen and that women who suffer from the loss of vaginal muscle tone will benefit most from Kegel exercises, while others feel that estrogen will strengthen the muscles in the pelvic area and can help with stress urinary incontinence, or the loss of urine when you laugh, sneeze, or cough. In addition to its possible effect on vaginal muscles, estrogen replacement causes the urethra to develop a healthier and thicker mucous lining and surrounding tissues, and, as a result, urinary infections will be less frequent.

Skin Changes

Estrogen makes the skin retain more water so that fine skin lines become less visible. It also helps maintain the collagen that keeps skin looking moist. It does not prevent wrinkles.

Mood Changes

Estrogen can help with mood changes. Some of the mood changes you may experience are due to insomnia and night sweats. Because estrogen therapy provides relief from hot flashes and night sweats, it can ease the anxiety or insomnia caused by these problems. In addition, estrogen itself appears to improve the quality of sleep, in that it increases the time you spend in rapid-eye-movement (REM) sleep, which is the stage of sleep associated with dreaming.

Some mood changes you may experience are not related to insomnia. For example, many menopausal women report having feelings of anxiety, depression, listlessness, and headaches. These symptoms are not necessarily related to hormone changes, but they do tend to lessen with the use of HRT. If you have a serious depression, however, HRT may make you feel even more depressed. Psychotherapy and the use of antidepressant medication are the treatment of choice for serious depressions. See chapter 10 for further information.

Heart Disease

Women appear to be relatively protected from heart disease until menopause. Ten to fifteen years after menopause, however, they share the same risk of heart disease as men; it is the number one cause of death in women over the age of forty.

If you are protected from heart disease because of estrogen before menopause, can HRT provide the same protection after menopause? Most research to date indicates that estrogen supplements offer protection from heart disease. In nineteen major studies done before 1991, eleven found that women who took estrogen reduced the risk of heart disease by 50 percent or greater, four showed a risk reduction of 30 to 50 percent, and two reported no difference. Only two studies found an increased risk, and in one of those, the heart disease occurred mostly in women who were smokers and over the age of sixty.

The largest study to date, the Nurses' Health Study, was reported in the *New England Journal of Medicine* in 1991. It followed fifty thousand menopausal nurses, and found that the women who took estrogen decreased their incidence of heart attacks by 50 percent. Even women with a low risk of having a heart attack had a significant reduction in their incidence of heart disease when they were on estrogen.

The criticism that has been leveled against these studies is that they involve a selection bias, in that women who choose or are chosen to be on HRT tend to be upper middle class and relatively well educated. These women see their doctors more often because they are taking hormones, and they may be receiving more preventive care or advice about lifestyle changes during these visits, which can help reduce the risk of heart disease.

Additional studies indicate that estrogen can have a positive influence on some of the factors that contribute to heart disease, such as serum lipid levels, blood clots, and blood vessel dilation. On the other hand, HRT may increase triglycerides. Triglycerides are fat molecules in the bloodstream that are frequently measured with cholesterol. However, the association of increased triglycerides and the risk of heart disease is less clear than it is with cholesterol. More research will help to clarify the effects of HRT on heart disease, and will eventually allow researchers to develop treatments with similar effects for women who cannot or choose not to take estrogen.

Osteoporosis

Most researchers agree that taking estrogen can prevent or greatly reduce bone loss after menopause and therefore reduce the risk of bone fractures. To be effective in this way, HRT must begin within six years after menopause, since half of the bone that is lost after menopause will occur within the first seven years. If you begin HRT later, significant bone loss may have already occurred and you will be less protected against the development of fractures. HRT does not help you build bone. It merely stops the acceleration of the bone loss.

Once you stop HRT, you will continue to lose bone at the same rate as if you had never been on it. Thus, HRT is a long-term commitment if you hope to reduce the risk of osteoporosis. You will have to stay on HRT until bone loss slows down naturally, which is around the age of sixty-five.

Colon Cancer

A large study released in April 1995 found that estrogen users had a 29 percent lower risk of dying from colon cancer than nonusers. For those who had been on estrogen for more than ten years, the risk was 55 percent lower.

Mental Deterioration

Several small trials have indicated that estrogen improves memory for post-menopausal women. In 1993, another study found that HRT helped women with mild to moderate symptoms of Alzheimer's disease.

Side Effects of Hormone Replacement Therapy

There are various side effects that can occur as the result of the use of hormones. Some of these are more common than others, and some are more tolerable than others.

Table 6.2
Common Side Effects of Estrogen

These side effects are unpleasant and may make you uncomfortable enough to discontinue estrogen:

- Breast tenderness or enlargement

- Enlargement of fibroids (rare)

- Spotty darkening of the skin, particularly on the neck and chest

- Fluid retention

Common Side Effects of Progestins

These side effects are similar to the symptoms seen with PMS:

- Breast tenderness
- Irritability
- Weight gain
- Lower abdominal pressure
- Constipation
- Fluid retention
- Increased appetite
- Depression
- Acne

Because the most common reason why women discontinue HRT is the vaginal bleeding that can occur with progestin, it should be noted that millions of women have taken progestin with no serious side effects and there are no known long-term negative effects. Progestin protects women from developing endometrial cancer, although it is not approved by the Food and Drug Administration (FDA) for this particular use. Side effects may be less likely with natural progesterone.

Risks of Hormone Replacement Therapy

Endometrial Cancer

The latest data released by the PEPI Study (Postmenopausal Estrogen/Progestin Intervention Study), published in the February 1996 edition of the *Journal of the American Medical Association*, revealed that women who had taken estrogen alone had a high rate of *endometrial hyperplasia*, a condition in which the lining of the uterus grows excessively. Hyperplasia is considered a precursor of cancer. In addition, women who had taken estrogen alone had more unscheduled biopsies, required significantly more D & Cs, and had a slightly increased rate of hysterectomy compared to the groups who were taking a combination of estrogen and progesterone.

The current recommendation is that if you take estrogen alone, your uterine lining will need to be monitored annually. Unopposed estrogen therapy (estrogen without progesterone), however, can be used in women who have had a hysterectomy, since women without a uterus do not need progesterone.

Breast Cancer

While some early studies found links between estrogen and breast cancer, others have not, and the issue is still being debated. The latest results from the Nurses' Health Study, published in the 1995 *New England Journal of Medicine*, showed that the short-term use of hormones was not associated with an increase in breast cancer. The type of hormone regimen (estrogen alone or estrogen/progesterone) did not have a significant impact on the risk of developing breast cancer. However, a woman's age and the length of time she took hormones did. Breast cancer risk increased 40 percent in women ages fifty to sixty-four and 70 percent in women ages sixty-five to sixty-nine who were on hormone replacement therapy for more than five years.

While these numbers may sound frightening, it helps to look at it from a different perspective: A sixty-year-old woman who has used estrogen for at least five years has a 3 percent chance of developing breast cancer over the next five years, compared to a 1.8 percent chance for a woman who has not been on hormones. If hormones were taken for five years or less, excess risk disappeared. This risk drops to normal levels when a woman has been off of hormones for two years.

Gallbladder Disease

Women who take oral estrogen are more likely to develop gallbladder disease and gallstones requiring surgery than those who do not. At highest risk are women who are

Table 6.3
Effects of HRT on Breast Cancer Risk

Probability of breast cancer diagnosis this year

Your current age	With more than 5 years HRT	With 5 or fewer years HRT
50-54	1 in 320	1 in 450
55-59	1 in 276	1 in 386
60-64	1 in 209	1 in 292
65-69	1 in 144	1 in 244

Source: *New England Journal of Medicine,* June 15, 1995. Cancer Statistics Review 1973–1989.

overweight and have had several children. *Transdermal* (patch) estrogens may prevent the development of gall stones, since they bypass the liver.

Asthma

A recent report from the Nurses' Health Study suggests the risk of developing asthma increased by 50 percent in women who were currently taking estrogen. The longer the use and the higher the dose of estrogen, the greater their risk of developing asthma. If you have asthma and are on hormone replacement therapy (and find your asthma worsening) you may want to talk to your physician.

In making the decision of whether to take hormones or not, you will want to consult with your physician and consider your own unique risk factors for heart disease, breast cancer, and osteoporosis. If you have a family history of osteoporosis, heart attack before the age of sixty, or elevated cholesterol or triglycerides levels, you will probably be more inclined toward using hormone therapy. If there is a family history of certain cancers, however, you may want to consider alternative forms of treatment (see chapter 7). Remember that the decision to take or not take hormones is not irrevocable and can always be reversed as new information becomes available. If you choose to discontinue the use of hormones, it is recommended that you taper off slowly to minimize the return of menopausal changes.

Who Should Use Hormone Replacement Therapy with Caution?

Several conditions can worsen with cyclical estrogen. Caution should be used if you have

- Seizures
- Diabetes
- Migraine headaches
- Gallbladder disease
- Liver disease
- Asthma

You should **definitely not** take estrogen if you have:

- Endometrial cancer
- A history of breast cancer
- Unexplained vaginal bleeding

Most physicians feel that women who have breast cancer should not take estrogen because many breast cancers have estrogen receptors, and the introduction of estrogen could make tumors grow faster. However, there are many women who have survived breast cancer and are now at risk for developing coronary heart disease and osteoporosis. HRT in this group of women can be beneficial, but, again, there is controversy about whether this group of women should have HRT or not. This issue will have to be decided with further research. For women who are at increased risk for developing cancer, tamoxifen (Nolvadex), which

---

Table 6.4
Summary of Benefits and Risks of Estrogen Replacement Therapy

Proven benefits	**Likely benefits**
• Relieves Hot Flashes	• Reduces risk of heart disease
• Relieves vaginal dryness and atrophy	• Helps the skin retain more water
• Reduces bone loss	• Diminishes mood changes
Proven risks	**Likely risks**
• Increases risk of endometrial cancer (unless used in conjunction with progestin)	• Can aggravate seizures, diabetes, migraines, asthma, and liver disease
• May increase the risk of gallstones	• May cause blood clots
• May increase growth of fibroid tumors in the uterus	• May increase the risk of breast cancer

acts like estrogen on the heart and bones and an antiestrogen on breast tissue, can be used. The research is continuing to evolve on the optimal length of treatment with tamoxifen. It is important to confer with your physician to learn the latest results of the medical studies as they are published.

If You Decide to Take Hormones, Which Kind Do You Take?

Estrogen

The most commonly used estrogen is *Premarin,* a mixture of estrogens derived from the urine of pregnant mares that comes in pill form. It has been the most widely studied compound for its ability to relieve menopausal changes. While there is not adequate information to determine whether the other available oral estrogens are equivalent to Premarin, any of the other estrogens on the market are effective in relieving menopausal symptoms.

Oral estrogens are digested and pass through the liver, where they are broken down, before entering the blood stream. In general, conjugated and esterified estrogens, which are fairly large molecules, are more likely to get through the liver intact. They are more potent because they leave more estrogen intact than micronized estrogens. While in the liver, estrogen stimulates the production of certain proteins that may increase the risk of blood clots in a few women. It also stimulates the liver to make cholesterol. While most of the cholesterol produced is the good cholesterol (HDL), increased levels of cholesterol can cause gallbladder problems.

Different preparations of estrogen may be tolerated better by some women, and therefore, may be useful alternatives to Premarin. Esterified estrogen compounds (Estratab) are similar to Premarin but have a different combination of estrogens. Estradiol, the predominant estrogen in premenopausal women, is available as a pill (Estrace) or a skin patch (Estraderm or Climara). It may be used for women who are experiencing premature menopause. If the patch is used, it is applied to the abdomen or buttocks and is changed every three days with Estraderm, or once a week with Climara. Because the estrogen is absorbed through the skin, it passes directly through the bloodstream and enters the liver in much lower concentrations. By avoiding the liver, this preparation may reduce the risk of gallstones and blood clots. However, since the estrogen will not go through the liver, it may not affect cholersterol levels as much.

Estrogen is also available as a cream, which has been effective in relieving vaginal dryness. The estrogen in this preparation is absorbed into the body as well, but in varying amounts. The beneficial effects on heart and bone are not known.

Several products are available that combine estrogens and androgens (male hormones). Estratest is occasionally prescribed for women whose ovaries are removed before midlife. It is also used when women are troubled by the loss of libido that can accompany menopause. There are several reports that suggest that androgens will improve sexual desire. However, they can cause acne and excessive facial and body hair. Excessive levels can cause balding, upper body weight gain, a lowered voice, and clitoral enlargement. Their influence on heart disease is uncertain.

Most women beginning HRT are started on Premarin. The disadvantage of this method is that a constant level of estrogen may not always be maintained, so if you take the medication in the morning, you may experience hot flashes at night. This can be solved by dividing the dose of medication or taking the medication at night so that you can sleep. If you develop side effects due to a certain preparation, you can work with your doctor and switch to a different type of estrogen. Because each estrogen preparation is different and because women have different amounts of circulating estrogen and metabolize it differently, an individualized schedule is important.

Three major hormone replacement schedules are used. They are summarized in table 6.5. For women who have had a hysterectomy, estrogen can be taken alone without the use of progesterone. Unopposed estrogen therapy is not usually recommended for women who have a uterus because of the increased risk of endometrial cancer. If you are against taking progesterone and begin unopposed estrogen treatment, you should have a pretreatment endometrial biopsy and biopsies on a yearly basis. Experiencing any bleeding would be an indication for another endometrial biopsy.

Estrogen and progesterone in combination can be taken either cyclically or continuously. If you take estrogen cyclically, this more or less copies the natural menstrual cycle. Estrogen is taken on days one to twenty-five and progesterone is added on or about day fourteen. After day twenty-five, no hormone is taken for five days, during which time bleeding will probably occur. This bleeding gradually diminishes over the years and eventually disappears.

If you take estrogen and progesterone continuously, they are both taken every day. The lining of the uterus thins and never builds up, so there is no bleeding. However, because taking progesterone does not duplicate the cyclical biological schedule of the premenopausal woman, some researchers feel that it is less effective in protecting you against heart disease.

In using estrogens, you start with the lowest dose, 0.625 mg of Premarin or 1 mg of estradiol, or 0.5 mg if you are using the patch. If you still have hot flashes or irregular bleeding, speak to your doctor about it because your medication may need to be adjusted.

You can also use natural estrogens, derived from wild Mexican yams and soybeans. These preparations are associated with a lower incidence of side effects. They come as capsules, sublingual tablets, and creams. However, you would need to work with your doctor to find the correct dose. The ability of these substances to protect the heart and bones has not yet been studied.

Table 6.5
Hormone Replacement Schedules

Unopposed Estrogen: Continuous

Day of month	1 30
Estrogen	1 30
Progesterone	None
Bleeding	None
Pill:	0.625 mg estrogen or 1 mg estradiol
Patch:	0.05 or 0.1 mg

This is used in women who have had a hysterectomy. It is not recommended in women who still have a uterus because of the increased risk of endometrial cancer.

Cyclic Combined Schedule

Day of month	1 30
Estrogen	1 25
Progesterone	14. 25
Bleeding	25 30
Pill:	0.625 mg estrogen or 1 mg estradiol on days 1–25; 5 mg oral progestin on days 14–25
Patch:	0.05 or 0.1 mg estrogen plus 5 mg oral progestin

Continuous Combined Schedule

Day of month	1 30
Estrogen	1 30
Progesterone	1 30
Bleeding	Spotting can occur for up to one year
Pill:	0.625 mg estrogen or 1 mg estradiol plus 2.5 mg oral progestin
	or
Patch:	0.05 or 0.1 mg estrogen plus 2.5 mg oral progestin

Progesterone

The PEPI Study highlighted the superior effects of natural progesterone. Compared to the synthetic progesterone that is currently on the market (Provera), the natural progesterone was more effective in increasing HDL levels. In addition, there were fewer side effects, such as fluid retention, breast tenderness, and depression. However, natural progesterone is not currently widely available in the United States. In Europe it is available as Utrogestan, produced by Besins-Isovesco. Some druggists are making their own versions, and several mail-order pharmacies are offering natural progesterone pills, tablets, and suppositories by prescription.

Finding the right type of hormone replacement therapy, both in terms of dosage and preparation, should be individualized. How long you stay on hormones should also be individualized. Knowing that it may take several trials of different preparations before you find the one with which you are most comfortable can also help you persist in taking medication if you encounter unpleasant side effects.

You must maintain a relationship with your physician, who will take a family history, along with giving a pelvic examination, Pap smear, breast exam, and blood tests to measure cholesterol, blood sugar, hormone levels, and calcium levels. She or he may also order a mammogram, bone density survey, electrocardiogram, and a test to examine the lining of your uterus. Follow-up visits will vary.

In the end, the decision to take hormones is a very personal choice. The American College of Obstetricians and Gynecologists offers the following advice to its practitioners:

> *At present, there are insufficient data to indicate that all postmenopausal women must be treated with estrogen replacement. For that reason, the benefits and risks, as they pertain to each patient, should be reviewed with her in detail. Ultimately, it is the patient who must decide and give her informed consent.*

Summary

The decision to take hormones is a personal one. In order to make a choice, the following questions may be helpful:

- What are the pros and cons of HRT?

- How disabling are the changes you are having with menopause? You can use the Menopausal Distress Severity chart in chapter 3 to determine this.

- Do you have heart disease or risk factors for heart disease?

- Do you have osteoporosis or risk factors for osteoporosis?

- Do you have or have you had breast cancer?

- How concerned are you about endometrial cancer?

Table 6.6
Options for HRT

Trade name	Generic	Source	Comments
Estrogens:			
Oral			
Premarin	Conjugated equine estrogens	Urine of pregnant mares	Most widely studied
Estratab, Menest	Esterified estrogens	Modified soy estrogens	Thought to be as effective as Premarin
Estrace	Estradiol	Natural plant compound	Requires higher dose than other estrogens
Ogen, Ortho-est	Estrone estropipate	Modified plant estrogen	Thought to be less potent than Premarin
Patches			
Estraderm, Climara, Vivelle	Estradiol	Natural plant compound	Bypasses liver so does not raise HDL
Progestogens:			
Oral			
Provera, Cycrin	Medroxyprogest- erone acetate (MPA)	Synthesized from plants	Most widely studied; generic form available
Aygestin	Norethindrone acetate	Derived from synthetic androgens	May lower HDL substantially
Prometrium	Micronized progesterone	Natural plant compound	Fewer systemic side effects than MPA
Intrauterine			
Progestasert	Micronized progesterone	Natural plant compound	Fewer systemic side effects; must replace annually
Combinations:			
Prempro	Conjugated estro- gens and MPA	Premarin/MPA	Single pill combination
Premphase	Conjugated estro- gens and MPA	Premarin/MPA	Single pill cyclic regimen
Estratest	Esterified estrogens and methyltestosterone	Plant-derived synthetics	May boost libido; long-term effects unknown

Source: *Harvard Women's Health Watch*, May 1996.

The Decision to Take Hormones

	None	Mild	Moderate	Severe
How disabling are your menopausal changes? (from table 3.3)				

Do you have:	Yes	No
Heart disease?	_____	_____
Risk factors for heart disease?	_____	_____
Osteoporosis?	_____	_____
Risk factors for osteoporosis?	_____	_____
Breast cancer?	_____	_____
Are you concerned about endometrial cancer?	_____	_____
Do you have a family history of:		
Cancer?	_____	_____
Heart Disease?	_____	_____
Osteoporosis?	_____	_____
Do you have medical conditions that make HRT inadvisable?	_____	_____
Are you willing to take medication regularly?	_____	_____
Have you considered alternatives to HRT?	_____	_____
Are you willing to:		
Eat well?	_____	_____
Exercise regularly?	_____	_____
Stop smoking?	_____	_____
Maintain a desirable weight?	_____	_____
Keep cholesterol under control?	_____	_____
Keep blood pressure under control?	_____	_____
Maintain low caffeine and alcohol intake?	_____	_____

After you have answered these questions for yourself, you will be in a better position to discuss HRT with your physician. Remember, any choice you make is not irrevocable and can be changed in the light of new research information or as alternative treatments become available.

- Do you have a family history of heart disease, osteoporosis, or breast cancer?

- Do you have a medical condition that makes taking HRT inadvisable?

- Are you familiar with the concept of risk described in appendix D?

- What are your attitudes toward heart disease, osteoporosis, and aging? In most cases where the evidence is not clearly on one side or the other, the final decision is often based on attitudes toward these issues.

- Are you willing to make lifestyle changes in exercise, diet, weight, cholesterol, blood pressure control, and cease smoking?

- Are you willing to take medication regularly?

- Have you considered alternatives to HRT? (See chapter 7.)

- What are your goals and what do you expect from HRT?

7

Alternatives to Hormone Replacement Therapy

Many people today seek nontraditional alternatives to HRT. Their reasons for seeking such treatments vary from a distrust of the conventional medical profession to a desire to focus on the whole person, rather than on one body system. There are many different types of nontraditional approaches. For the most part, these treatments have not been specifically designed for remedying menopausal changes. This chapter focuses on

- Herbs, foods, and supplements
- Acupuncture
- Homeopathy

Few of these treatments have been scientifically tested; however, this does not mean that they are ineffective or harmful. Nevertheless, before you try any of these approaches you should seek information about them from reputable, preferably licensed, sources. A number of helpful organizations are listed in appendix E.

Herbs, Foods, and Supplements

A recent edition of *Consumer Reports* (November 1995) states that the use of herbal remedies is growing by about 15 percent each year, and now totals almost half of the use of more traditional vitamins and minerals. Claims are made that these remedies can cure or prevent almost any malady. Nevertheless, it is important to be aware that claims can be made on packages with little, if any, evidence for safety or effectiveness. Since FDA approval is not needed, the supplements can be manufactured without adhering to any standards. *Consumer Reports* suggests that you seek information from independent sources and recommends two books that are listed in appendix E.

Because an herb or supplement may interact with another drug you are taking, or may have a side effect that could be serious, check with your doctor first. This is especially true for pregnant or nursing women, or those who have chronic or serious health problems.

Consumer Reports suggests

- Start with small doses.

- Check warnings on packages.

- Begin by using single herb products rather than combinations of herb products, so you can sort out the effects of each product.

Table 7.1
Herbs, Foods, and Supplements

Symptom	Herb
Hot flashes	Ginseng, Dong Quai, Black Cohosh, Blue Cohosh, Sarsaparilla, Licorice, Bioflavonoids, Evening Primrose Oil, False Unicorn Root, Fennel, Wild Mexican Yam, Soy Products
Fatigue	Ginseng, Blessed Thistle, Cayenne Pepper, Ginger, Oatstraw
Depression	Ginseng, Blessed Thistle, Cayenne Pepper, Ginger, Oatstraw
Anxiety	Valerian, Chamomile Tea, Passion Flower
Insomnia	Valerian
Vaginal dryness	Evening Primrose Oil, Vitamin E, Flax Seed Oil, Soy Products
Skin changes	Evening Primrose Oil, Flax Seed Oil
Osteoporosis	Wild Mexican Yam, Red Raspberry Leaf
Bleeding	Bioflavinoids

- Be objective about the effects, both positive and negative.

- If there is a problem, stop the supplement and call your physician.

- Remember that "natural" or "organic" does not necessarily mean "safe."

- Make sure the label states that the dosages of active ingredients have been standardized. (Since herbs are often used in these preparations, the concentration of active ingredients in each plant, and therefore in each dose, can differ significantly. When the label states that the dosage has been "standardized," the company has attempted to make sure that each dose contains the same amounts of active ingredients.)

Several sources list the herbs, foods, and supplements in table 7.1 as being frequently recommended for specific menopausal changes. Some of the herbs reportedly have estrogen-like or progesterone-like substances or precursors. As a result, some women's health problems may preclude use of these substances, for example, women with breast cancer. It is also important to remember that just because a supplement eases effects such as hot flashes, it may not provide the protection that estrogen does against heart disease and osteoporosis.

Acupuncture

Acupuncture has a long history of being used as anesthesia. It is believed to enhance the production of endorphins, which are natural morphine-like substances produced by the body. Acupuncture involves inserting very fine, stainless steel needles (sterilized and often disposable) at particular points in the body, and leaving them in place for approximately twenty minutes. It may take several treatments before any effect is noticed.

In addition to its effectiveness in controlling pain, there are reports that acupuncture can be helpful for

- Cystitis
- Menstrual Problems
- PMS
- Insomnia
- Headaches
- Anxiety
- Depression

Homeopathy

Homeopathy, which dates back to the late eighteenth century, is based on the premise that extremely diluted solutions could prevent symptoms that the same solution at higher doses could cause. Western medicine, in contrast, often practices *allopathy*, which means "opposite disease," where medications are given to produce the opposite state of the symptom.

There are up to fifteen different homeopathic remedies used for treating menopausal changes. It may take four to five weeks to determine the effectiveness, and you may develop a temporary increase in your symptoms before they decrease. The total process may take as long as a year or two and it is recommended that you work with a licensed practioner. Again, as with herbal remedies, these treatments may not provide any long-term protection against heart disease or osteoporosis. Table 7.2 includes some of the more commonly prescribed homeopathic remedies.

Refer to appendix E for information on homeopathy and acupuncture resources.

Table 7.2
Homeopathic Remedies

For Hot Flashes	For Vaginal Dryness
Sulfur	Nat Mur
Sepia	Bryonia
Lachesis	Staphisagria
Belladonna	
Pulsatilla	

Summary

- While alternative remedies and techniques may be useful, many are unproven by Western standards, and some might be dangerous.

- If you choose to pursue these treatments, be informed and seek qualified practitioners.

- Try one herb, supplement, or remedy at a time, so you can objectively evaluate the results.

- If you have any negative effects, stop the treatment and speak to your physician.

- If you use these approaches and are not using HRT, close medical supervision is strongly suggested to prevent and monitor osteoporosis and heart disease.

8

Lifestyle Changes

In this chapter, the following lifestyle changes, which can have a positive impact on both your physical and emotional well-being during the menopausal years, will be explored

- Exercise

- Nutrition

- Alcohol

- Caffeine

- Smoking

Exercise

The importance of exercise in your life cannot be overemphasized, and it is never too early or too late to begin. When it is part of your weekly routine, exercise improves almost every aspect of life. Research has shown that even nursing home residents can benefit by beginning an exercise program!

How to Begin

Before beginning any exercise program, it is important to check it out with your physician. Once you've done that, it is beneficial to have a basic knowledge about exercise.

Advantages of Exercise

- Appropriate exercise may help add and maintain calcium in the bones, hence decreasing the development of osteoporosis. This is especially important if you are not taking hormone replacement therapy.

- Regular aerobic exercise, in conjunction with a healthy diet, significantly decreases the risk of heart disease by raising the levels of high density lipoproteins (HDLs), the good cholesterol.

- Exercise helps control weight by

    1. Causing more calories to be burnt post-exercise

    2. Reducing your appetite

    3. Creating more calorie-using muscle mass

- By increasing endorphin production, exercise can help boost your mood and moderate your stress.

- Exercise can enrich your sex life, through improved mood management and stress reduction, as well as increased fitness, energy, endurance, and motivation.

There are three areas to focus on in developing a well-rounded exercise program: building *strength* (and maintaining calcium in the bones), *endurance* (cardiovascular fitness), and *flexibility*. All of these areas should be included in your program.

Strength building occurs to some extent with almost all forms of exercise. However, many cardiovascular and most flexibility exercises either do not stress the skeletal system enough to preserve calcium on the bone, or will only work certain muscles. Cycling, for example, builds strength in the lower body and is cardiovascular, but it does not provide much resistance for the bones, nor does it offer much exercise for the upper body. In this case, a well-rounded program would also need to include strength-building exercises for the upper body and exercises that provide resistance for the bones.

When exercise is discussed in regard to the prevention of osteoporosis, the term "weight-bearing" is often used. That term, however, may be a bit misleading because you can assume it means exercise done while standing. That is not necessarily true. More research about exercise and the prevention of osteoporosis is still needed before definitive statements can be made. However, it seems that in order for exercise to be effective in preventing bone loss, the skeleton needs to be at least moderately stressed, that is, the skeleton must "bear weight," although not to the point where injury can occur. The National Osteoporosis Foundation cautiously (because of the paucity of research) recommends the following:

- Running or jogging
- Aerobics
- Weight training
- Stair climbing
- Racquet sports
- Field sports (e.g., field hockey, soccer)
- Court sports (e.g., volleyball, basketball)
- Dancing (e.g., folk, square, ballet)

Recommendations about frequency, intensity, and duration of exercise to prevent osteoporosis are also not clear-cut, but many authorities suggest doing the activity at least three days per week for twenty to thirty minutes. While activities such as swimming and walking have not been consistently associated with increased bone mass, these forms of exercise may help to decrease the overall risk of osteoporosis by enhancing balance and aerobic capacity. There are no data about activities such as cycling or skiing. Like swimming and walking, however, these activities can enhance balance and aerobic capacity.

Table 8.1
Recommended Heart Rates During Exercise*

Age	Maximum	65% of max.	85% of max.
20	200	130	170
25	195	127	166
30	190	124	162
35	185	120	157
40	180	117	153
45	175	114	149
50	170	111	145
55	165	107	140
60	160	104	136
65+	150	98	128

*Based on resting heart rate of 72 for males and 80 for females. Men over forty and people with any heart problem should have a stress electrocardiogram before starting an exercise program.

Cardiovascular, or *aerobic* (meaning "with oxygen") *exercise,* is the form of exercise most beneficial to the heart. It requires uninterrupted activity for at least twenty minutes or more, three to five times a week. During this activity, your heart rate must remain between 65 percent and 85 percent of its maximum (see table 8.1). Again, be sure to get checked by your physician first, especially if you have any history of heart problems.

Table 8.2
How Many Calories Do You Burn?
Calories Used Per Minute According to Your Weight

Weight in Pounds

Activity	100	120	150	170	200	220	250
Anaerobic	**Calories Burned**						
Calisthenics	3.3	3.9	4.9	5.6	6.6	7.2	8.2
Golf	3.6	4.3	5.4	6.1	7.2	7.9	9.0
Racquetball	6.3	7.6	9.5	10.7	12.7	13.9	15.8
Skiing, Downhill	6.3	7.6	9.5	10.7	12.7	13.9	15.8
Tennis	4.5	5.4	6.8	7.7	9.1	10.0	11.4
*Aerobic**							
Bicycling, 5.5 mph	3.1	3.8	4.7	5.3	6.3	6.9	7.9
Bicycling, 10 mph	5.4	6.5	8.1	9.2	10.8	11.9	13.6
Jogging, 11-min. mile	6.1	7.3	9.1	10.4	12.2	13.4	15.3
Running, 8-min. mile	9.4	11.3	14.1	16.0	18.8	20.7	23.5
Skiing, cross-country	7.2	8.7	10.8	12.3	14.5	15.9	18.0
Swimming, crawl stroke	5.8	6.9	8.7	9.8	11.6	12.7	14.5
Walking, 3 mph	2.7	3.2	4.0	4.6	5.4	5.9	6.8
Walking, 4 mph	3.9	4.6	5.8	6.6	7.8	8.5	9.7

*Note: Although these are continuous activities, your heart rate must remain within your target zone for the duration of the exercise to give aerobic benefit.

Many different types of exercise qualify as aerobic, including:

- Jogging
- Brisk walking
- Swimming
- Bicycling
- Cross-country skiing
- Stair-climbing
- Rowing
- Aerobic dance
- Water exercise

Today, many low- or nonimpact aerobic classes and tapes exist that will significantly reduce your risk of injury while providing you with the cardiovascular benefits you are seeking. If you use an instructor or personal trainer, make sure he or she is competent, knowledgeable, and able to work with you on your goals. Do not continue with an instructor or class that encourages you to do anything that is painful or about which you're unsure. Also remember that, whatever form of exercise you choose, a warm-up and cooldown are essential to prevent injury.

Table 8.2 shows you how many calories you will burn doing aerobic and anaerobic exercises. These numbers are estimates, because the more a person weighs, the more calories they require to do any activity. In addition, the vigor with which each person exercises will influence the number of calories burned.

Exercise Tips

- Schedule your exercise so that it is convenient and fits with your lifestyle. Look at chapters 10, 11, and 12, on mood and stress management, for examples of different types of exercise schedules.

- Vary your program. Variety makes exercise more interesting so that you will be more likely to continue to do it. Have a back-up plan for days when you're low on energy or time, or when the weather is bad.

- Whenever you say you can't afford the time to exercise, respond by saying, "I can't afford *not* to!"

- Start slowly. Five minutes of walking is a lot better than nothing.

- Work your way up (in terms of weight, time, and distance) gradually.

- Make exercise enjoyable. For example, exercise with a friend, or while listening to a book on tape.

Flexibility is the third component of exercise and can be achieved by slow, gentle stretches during your warm-up and cooldown. It is important not to bounce while doing these exercises. Yoga is a good flexibility builder and offers the additional benefit of relaxation.

Nutrition

Good nutrition is especially important for women in the menopausal years. For comprehensive information on nutrition, consult a good sourcebook, such as *Jane Brody's Nutrition Book* (see appendix E).

General Nutrition and Weight Loss

As you age, your metabolism slows and, for women who do not use estrogen, the risk of heart disease increases. For these reasons, it is important to eat a diet low in fat and

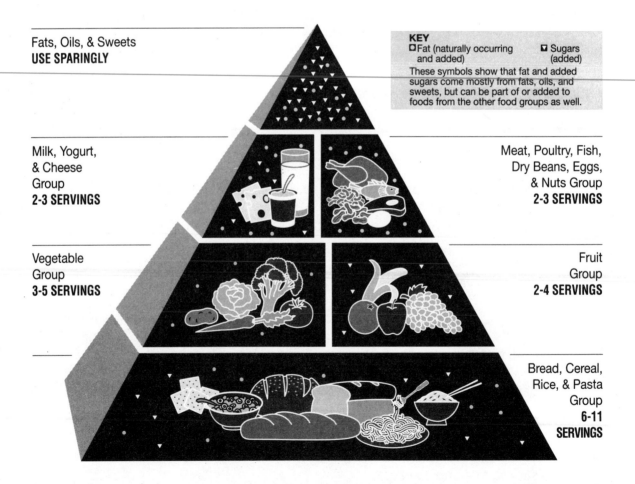

Fats, Oils, & Sweets
USE SPARINGLY

KEY
☐ Fat (naturally occurring and added)   ☑ Sugars (added)
These symbols show that fat and added sugars come mostly from fats, oils, and sweets, but can be part of or added to foods from the other food groups as well.

Milk, Yogurt, & Cheese Group
2-3 SERVINGS

Meat, Poultry, Fish, Dry Beans, Eggs, & Nuts Group
2-3 SERVINGS

Vegetable Group
3-5 SERVINGS

Fruit Group
2-4 SERVINGS

Bread, Cereal, Rice, & Pasta Group
6-11 SERVINGS

Sources: Food Pyramid provided by the National Center for Nutrition and Dietetics of the American Dietetic Association, Chicago, IL.

Nutrition Tips

- Make small dietary changes. If you decrease your food intake by 100 calories per day from your maintenance level (preferably fat calories) and make no other changes, you will lose *10 pounds* over the course of a year.

- Replace high-fat foods with low- or nonfat substitutes. For example, lowfat mayonnaise, nonfat yogurt, and nonfat sour cream will save you many fat calories and you will still feel satisfied.

- Most fast-food franchises now offer salads and other lowfat alternatives that are very convenient and tasty.

- Set realistic goals for weight. Do not expect to weigh exactly what you did when you were twenty. Focus on staying at a healthy weight, rather than an unrealistic one.

- Guard against being too thin. Thin people have a higher risk for osteoporosis, and must pay special attention to calcium, exercise, and hormone replacement therapy.

- Drink 6 to 8 glasses of water a day.

- Reduce salt and sugar. Sugar has "empty calories" in that it does not supply much nutrition. Salt can complicate hypertension, as well as make you retain fluid, creating feelings of bloatedness. Since both are acquired tastes, as you decrease their use, you will experience fewer cravings for them.

- If you are struggling with weight or nutrition, it may be helpful to consult a registered dietician.

high in fiber and complex carbohydrates throughout your adult years. No more than 25 to 30 percent of your calories should come from fat and, of that, as little from sources of saturated fat as possible. This type of diet can decrease your risk of certain types of cancer, and can also have a positive influence on hot flashes. Only 10 to 15 percent of your daily calories should come from protein. The remainder (55 to 65 percent) should come from complex carbohydrates.

Vitamins and Minerals

Although experts recommend you try to obtain all of the vitamins and minerals required for good health in a well-balanced diet, this becomes more difficult with age. As you get older, your body requires fewer calories. As a result, you often eat less. This means you're being asked to get more nutrition from less food every year. Because of this, a daily multivitamin and mineral supplement is often recommended. However, too much of a good thing isn't always healthy. Megadoses of certain vitamins, especially the fat-soluble vitamins

Healthy Weights for Women

Height	Weight
4'10"	91–119 lbs.
4'11"	94–122 lbs.
5'0"	96–125 lbs.
5'1"	99–128 lbs.
5'2"	102–131 lbs.
5'3"	105–134 lbs.
5'4"	108–138 lbs.
5'5"	111–142 lbs.
5'6"	114–146 lbs.
5'7"	118–150 lbs.
5'8"	122–154 lbs.
5'9"	126–158 lbs.
5'10"	130–163 lbs.
5'11"	134–168 lbs.
6'0"	138–173 lbs.

Source: U.S. Department of Health, Education, and Welfare.

(for example, A, D, and E) can be dangerous. Even the water-soluble vitamins, including vitamin C, can cause problems if taken in very large quantities.

Many supplements are *antioxidants*. These are substances thought to help prevent or slow down some cancers and other aspects of aging. Antioxidants include vitamins C, E, and beta-carotene (a precursor of vitamin A). Good natural sources of beta-carotene include dark green leafy vegetables (such as spinach), "yellow" vegetables (such as carrots and sweet potatoes), and orange fruits (such as cantaloupe). Recent research suggests that vitamin E, when taken over the long run, may significantly reduce the incidence of heart attacks. However, this research was done with men and may not apply to women.

Other recent findings strongly contradict previous studies which suggested that beta-carotene might be helpful in reducing the risk of lung cancer in smokers. As with all research regarding health, new data arise regularly, and it is very important to keep up to date.

Table 8.3
Calcium-Rich Foods

Item	Serving size	Calcium (mg)
Yogurt, plain lowfat	1 cup	415
Sardines, with bones	3 ounces	372
Ricotta, part skim	1/2 cup	337
Skim milk	1 cup	302
Whole milk	1 cup	291
Swiss cheese	1 ounce	262
Cheddar cheese	1 ounce	213
American cheese	1 ounce	198
Oysters	3/4 cup	170
Salmon, canned with bones	3 ounces	167
Collard greens	1/2 cup	145
Spinach, cooked	1/2 cup	106
Mustard greens, cooked	1/2 cup	97
Corn muffin	2 medium	90
Ice cream	1/2 cup	88
Cottage cheese, 2 percent fat	1/2 cup	77
Kale, cooked	1/2 cup	74
Broccoli, cooked	1/2 cup	68

Source: U.S. Department of Agriculture.

Calcium

Because of the crucial role calcium plays in the prevention of osteoporosis, you should be taking in about 1500 mg per day if you are postmenopausal, and 1000 mg per day if you are premenopausal. If you can't get enough from food sources, you can use a calcium supplement with vitamin D, which aids in calcium absorption.

Iron-Rich Foods

- Potatoes
- Red meats
- Enriched and whole grain cereals
- Dried fruit (raisins, apricots, and prunes)
- Liver (especially pork, followed by calf, beef, and chicken)

- Kidneys
- Green, leafy vegetables
- Dried beans and peas
- Blackstrap molasses
- Egg yolks

Iron

During the perimenopausal years, menstrual bleeding can become quite excessive, causing you to lose a lot of iron. Symptoms of iron-deficiency anemia include fatigue, weakness, paleness, and shortness of breath. Eating iron-rich foods, such as those listed below, can be a helpful, preventive measure. If that is not sufficient or possible, your doctor may prescribe iron supplements.

Fiber

Fiber refers to substances that primarily come from the cell walls of plants. Most fiber passes through the body undigested, but it is extremely important for a variety of reasons:

- It provides a feeling of fullness without extra fat or calories.
- It acts as a natural laxative.
- It may help relieve hemorrhoids and diverticular disease.
- It may help reduce the risk of colon cancer.
- It may also help reduce the risk of breast cancer.
- Certain types of fiber appear to lower cholesterol levels in the blood (pectins—found mostly in fruit, guar gum—found in beans, and the fiber found in oats, bran, and carrots).
- It can have a beneficial effect on blood sugar levels for diabetics.

Increase your fiber intake, gradually, to about 40 grams per day. Be wary that too much fiber can interfere in the absorption of other nutrients. Also, be sure to drink lots of water when you eat fiber, to prevent constipation. When you buy breads and cereals, be sure to read the label and look for the words "whole grain." Be mindful that because different types of fiber serve different health needs, it is important to get your fiber from a variety of food sources. Get your physician's advice prior to making any significant change in health

Dietary Fiber in Your Food

Food	Serving size	Weight (g)	Fiber (g)
Breads and Crackers			
Graham crackers	2 squares	15	1.5
Whole-wheat bread	1 slice	25	2.4
Cereals and Grains			
All-Bran or 100% Bran	1 cup	70	23.0
Grape-Nuts	1/3 cup	45	5.0
Rice, brown, cooked	1 cup	65	1.1
Rice, white, cooked	1 cup	65	0.4
Rolled oats, dry	1/2 cup	50	4.5
Shredded wheat	2 biscuits	50	6.1
Fruits			
Apple	1 small	90	3.1
Applesauce	1/2 cup	120	1.7
Banana	1 medium	100	1.8
Cantaloupe, cubes	3/4 cup	120	1.4
Grapefruit 1/2		200	2.6
Grapes, raw	16	60	0.4
Peach, raw	1 medium	100	1.3
Pear, raw	1 medium	120	2.8
Pears, canned	1/2 cup	125	1.4
Strawberries	1/2 cup	125	2.6
Vegetables			
Beans, green	1/2 cup	50	1.2
Broccoli, cooked	3/4 cup	75	1.6
Carrots, cooked	3/4 cup	100	2.1
Carrots, raw	1 medium	100	3.7
Cauliflower, raw	1 cup	100	1.8
Celery, raw	2-1/2 stalks	100	3.0
Corn kernels	2/3 cup	110	4.2
Cucumber	1/2 of 7-inch cucumber	100	1.5
Lettuce	1 cup	50	0.8
Spinach	2 large leaves	50	1.8
Summer squash, raw	1 5-inch squash	100	3.0

Source: The above fiber analyses were prepared by Dr. James W. Anderson, professor of medicine and clinical nutrition at the University of Kentucky Medical Center in Lexington, Kentucky.

habits, including nutrition. Use the list on the next page to help you make your dietary selections.

Soy Products

Recent research suggests that soy products can stimulate the production of estrogen. In 1988, a study of over a thousand Japanese women, ages forty-five to fifty-five, showed that they suffered from fewer hot flashes and other menopausal changes than women in Western cultures. It was believed that this was due to the high usage of soybean products in the Japanese diet.

In addition to being a source of natural estrogen, soy products (consumed in quantities of 25–50 grams a day) may also lower cholesterol levels, decrease levels of LDL, and increase levels of HDL. The plant estrogens in soy products may also protect against some hormone-related cancers.

Alcohol

Recent studies suggest that small amounts of alcohol, no more than one or two glasses of wine or beer per day, can have a protective effect on the heart. On the other hand, alcohol can

- Leach calcium

- Set off hot flashes

- Cause sleep disturbances

- Exacerbate depression

- Increase the risk of alcoholism

- Cause weight gain without providing any nutritional value

If alcohol is a problem for you, many organizations are available for free or low-cost assistance, such as Alcoholics Anonymous or Rational Recovery. See appendix E for more information.

Caffeine

In addition to coffee and tea, there are many other (often hidden) sources of caffeine. Many soft drinks have caffeine in them, even some clear soft drinks. Chocolate also has caffeine, as do some aspirin-type pain relievers. Caffeine can

- Increase the risk of fibrocystic breast disease

Tips to Stop Smoking

- Attend a support group (see the section on support groups in chapter 15 for information about how to access a group).

- Read a self-help book (see appendix E).

- Contact the American Lung Association for motivational information.

- Learn about other resources, such as the nicotine patch or gum, and ask your physician for a prescription if this is how you plan to quit.

- Reward, reward, reward! Reward yourself, on a daily basis, for every day that you've smoked fewer or no cigarettes.

- Consider whether "cold turkey" or a more gradual method will fit with your personality.

- Set realistic expectations for yourself.

- If you slip, it *doesn't* mean you've "blown" it (see chapter 11 for information on all-or-nothing thinking). Just get right back on track.

- Seek professional help from a therapist who specializes in smoking cessation.

- Set off hot flashes

- Increase anxiety

- Cause sleep disturbances

- Exacerbate osteoporosis

- Cause dehydration

If you would like to cut down on caffeine, do it gradually, as you might experience some "withdrawal symptoms," such as fatigue, irritability, or headaches.

Smoking

In a word, *don't.*

- Smoking can set off hot flashes.

- Smoking decreases the amount of estrogen in your system.

- Smoking can decrease bone mass and increase your risk of osteoporosis.

- Smoking increases your risk of heart disease and lung disease, lung cancer, breast cancer, bladder cancer, cervical cancer, and vulvar cancer

If you stop, or even decrease, your cigarette consumption now, you'll be doing great things for your health. So, how do you quit?

Summary

- There are a number of lifestyle changes you can make that will positively affect your physical and emotional well-being during menopause.

- Exercise can help your bones, heart, weight, and sex life.

- Beneficial nutritional changes can include changing your intake of fat, vitamins and minerals, and fiber.

- Moderating your alcohol intake can help with your bones, hot flashes, sleep, mood, and nutrition.

- Decreasing or eliminating smoking will provide tremendous benefits in many areas of health.

9

Sexuality

Menopause marks a change in your reproductive ability, but it does not mean the end of your sex life. This chapter will explore

- The effects on sexuality of biological changes in women at midlife
- The effects on sexuality of biological changes in men at midlife
- Loss of sexual interest
- Maximizing sexuality in midlife and beyond
- Other sexual problems that may occur
- Suggestions for coping with these changes and problems

A Woman's Sexual Response

To understand what happens because of aging and menopause, it is important to understand the normal sexual response. When you become sexually aroused, your pelvic area fills with blood and your vagina lubricates in anticipation of intercourse. The clitoris becomes enlarged as blood rushes into it. The upper part of the vagina lengthens and expands while the part nearest the vaginal opening becomes firm. During orgasm, rhythmic contractions of your uterus occur. After orgasm, there is a sense of physical relaxation. In this last phase of the arousal cycle, you will often be hypersensitive in your genital area and can be aroused again to experience additional orgasms.

As you age, you may find that it takes you longer to get aroused and that your arousal is less intense. After menopause, unless you have continued to be sexually active, it will take you longer to get lubricated, orgasms will be shorter, and uterine contractions will be less intense. The last phase of the arousal cycle will also be shorter. This is normal and to be expected.

Physical Changes Due to Menopause

One of the most important biological factors affecting your sexuality will be vaginal dryness, since vaginal lubrication decreases, or slows substantially, as estrogen decreases. The uterus and the cervix also become smaller, and, in some women, this may lead to painful uterine contractions during and after orgasm.

These changes may lead you to avoid intercourse, not because of a lack of desire, but because of the pain associated with it. These changes are very real, and can cause difficulties between you and your partner. The good news is that they are reversible with the use of estrogen or a topical ointment containing estrogen. Regular intercourse or masturbation can also help with vaginal dryness.

Loss of Sexual Interest

There is a great deal of variability in women's sexual responses at menopause. In the Stanford Menopause Study (1992), 71 percent of women noted changes in their interest in sex during perimenopause. Of them, 48 percent reported a marked decline in sexual interest, while 23 percent noticed an increase in libido. Another 20 percent reported that their interest in sex was unchanged. If a small decrease in sexual interest occurs, it may not feel problematic and you may not need to try to increase it. It will depend on how both you and your partner feel about it. It is not necessarily a sign of a physical or emotional problem, and doesn't necessarily reduce sexual fulfillment.

For those of you who experience a decline in sexual desire, its extent will depend, in part, on:

- Whether or not you have a current partner
- The quality of the relationship and communication with your current partner
- The level of your sex life prior to menopause (the more active you were before, the higher your sex drive is likely to be now)
- Fatigue level
- Sexual boredom
- The presence of other psychological problems, such as stress or depression
- The presence of other biological problems, such as vaginal dryness
- The use of certain medications, such as some medications for depression

Prescription for a Good Sex Life

- For biological changes associated with menopause (such as dryness) estrogen, used as a pill, patch, or cream, will provide a lot of relief.

- Regular sex is also very important for relieving vaginal dryness. Weekly intercourse or masturbation should be sufficient. The cliché, "use it or lose it," is accurate in this area.

- If lack of interest persists after alleviation of menopausal changes, low levels of testosterone may be the culprit. Usually, adequate amounts of testosterone are produced by the ovaries and adrenals. See table 9.1.

- The Kegel exercise not only decreases urinary incontinence, but it improves sexual functioning. It helps develop the muscles around the vagina, increasing your pleasure during sex. For more information, see chapter 4.

- For communication problems in relationships, learning and practicing communication skills are essential. For more information, see chapter 13.

- Communication can also help you and your partner understand the changes occurring in both of you and make adjustments to accommodate those changes.

- For relationship problems that are long-standing and unresolved, couples or marital counseling may be beneficial.

- Sex therapy, by a licensed therapist, can also be helpful. In this treatment, the therapist mostly focuses on education about sexuality, as well as on communication and suggestions about how to handle specific sexual problems between partners.

- For depression or other more serious psychological problems, such as a long-standing dislike of sex or previous sexual abuse, it will be important to get psychological help.

- Adding variety will help alleviate boredom, and may also help with physical or medical obstacles to sex that you or your partner may experience. In addition to intercourse, activities such as kissing, fondling, and caressing are important at any age.

- Masturbation is also normal and appropriate at any stage of the life cycle.

Table 9.1
Testosterone and Sex Drive in Women

Levels of testosterone of less than 30 nanograms per milliliter may be responsible for a woman's lack of sex drive. However, testosterone treatment remains controversial, and suitable doses and preparations of testosterone for this purpose are unknown. In anecdotal studies, women do report more desire when they take testosterone.

Testosterone can have the following side effects:

Positive Effects

- Relief from breast tenderness sometimes caused by HRT

Negative Effects

- Facial and chest hair
- Deepening of voice
- Acne
- Increased cholesterol

If you decide to try testosterone, be prepared for these potential side effects and the need for dosage adjustments.

Sex After Hysterectomy/Mastectomy

If you have had a hysterectomy that includes the removal of your ovaries, estrogen levels will fall precipitously. Hysterectomy can kill your sex drive. In addition, it can cause vaginal dryness, making intercourse unpleasant. Hysterectomy may also affect the quality of your orgasm because there will no longer be any uterine contractions. Some women may have feelings of being less attractive and desirable. Further, some men will treat women differently after hysterectomy.

Sex can also be affected after mastectomy. If the mastectomy has been for cancer, sex may be the last thing you have on your mind. In addition, if you have to have radiation or chemotherapy, the treatments may make you feel debilitated. Because so much of society's definition of a woman's attractiveness focuses on her appearance and her breasts, the loss of a breast can damage your self-image.

Here are some recommendations to help you in resuming sex after you have had a hysterectomy:

- Allow yourself a chance to heal.

- Use a mild lubricant, such as K-Y Jelly.

- Plan sexual activity for a time of day when your pain is least intense.

- Find a position for touching or intercourse that puts as little pressure as possible on the painful areas of your body.

- Focus on feelings of pleasure and excitement and not on pain.

- You may need help in dealing with the aftermath of surgery or radiation therapy. If you feel that you are not adjusting emotionally to the surgery, psychotherapy can be useful in helping you to restore your self-esteem and redefine your body image. Psychotherapy may also help if communication problems develop with your mate.

Contraception

During the perimenopausal and postmenopausal periods, the ovaries may produce an occasional egg. Because of this, birth control remains a necessity. You should continue to use contraception for a full year after your last menstrual period.

For the Newly Single

Some of you may be newly single, either as the result of divorce or widowhood. It can be scary, but also exhilarating, to begin dating again. However, you need to be aware of sexually transmitted diseases. The most common of these are caused by viruses and include HIV, herpes, and genital warts. Once you have contracted them, these viruses are relatively incurable. Of these, HIV infections almost always result in death. It is a good practice to use condoms in all sexual encounters: Do not have unprotected sex. Open communication with your partner about this topic is essential.

Physical Changes Occurring in Men

If your sexual partner is male, be aware that his sexual response is also likely to change in these ways as a result of aging:

- It takes longer to attain an erection.

- It may take more varied stimulation to attain an erection.

- It takes longer to reach ejaculation.

- Ejaculations are less forceful.

- The time between ejaculations is longer.

- Erections lose their firmness quickly after ejaculation.

If a man reacts to these changes with embarrassment, he may withdraw sexually from his partner, who in turn might misinterpret his withdrawal and feel that he is no longer interested in her. Tragically, this may set up a vicious cycle of insecurity, blame, and further withdrawal. Communication with your partner will help to prevent this. Other changes occurring in men are covered in chapter 14.

Summary

- Sex can continue to be pleasurable, no matter what your age.

- Normal changes occur in the female sexual response at menopause, including changes in lubrication and orgasm.

- You may experience a loss of sexual interest, which can be caused by a number of factors, including whether or not you have a partner and how active your sex life has been in the past.

- A decrease in sexual activity is not necessarily problematic. It depends on how both you and your partner feel about it.

- If you are having sexual problems, it is important to identify and treat them. There are a number of treatments available for a variety of problems.

- Regular sex, either by intercourse or masturbation, is helpful to maintain sexual function.

- Good communication with your partner enhances sex. See chapter 13 for more information.

- Men are also undergoing changes in their sexual response as a result of aging.

- Contraception should be used for a year after your last menstrual period.

10

Menopause and Mood

Although physical changes have occupied center stage so far in this book, the emotional issues and challenges encountered during menopause and midlife can also play a large role. Certainly the loss of fertility, in and of itself, can have emotional consequences. Many women are relieved at the prospect of no longer worrying about an unplanned pregnancy, and feel freer sexually, knowing they cannot become pregnant. However, even women who have never had a desire for children may feel sad at the loss of their fertility, since the decision not to have children is now final.

A number of other life events are commonly experienced during midlife, by both women and men, including

- Entry, re-entry, or exit from the workforce

- Change in job, career, or income

- Being a member of the "sandwich generation"— caring for family members in the older and younger generations simultaneously

- "Empty Nest" or "Return to the Nest"— coping with adult children who have left or returned home

- Becoming a grandparent

- Loss of a significant other or family member through death, divorce, or other circumstances

- Becoming single or entering new relationships

- Changes in appearance

- Concerns about illness and mortality

- Reevaluation of priorities

Each of these events can be challenging, even the positive changes, and is likely to require some adjustments. Many people will successfully meet these challenges, emerging with greater wisdom and an enhanced sense of self-confidence and self-acceptance. For some, however, there may be difficulties along the way, resulting in problems with depression or stress.

The next several chapters focus on understanding emotional reactions and learning how to deal with them, beginning with a look at mood. In the past, menopause and depression were thought to be inseparable. Physicians used the term "involutional melancholia" to describe depression that occurred at menopause. Women were, and still are in many cases, expected to become depressed, irritable, and anxious when they experience perimenopause and menopause. It is now known that this concept is largely untrue.

This chapter will discuss what depression is and is not. A clinically diagnosed serious depression is the most common emotional problem to affect women whether they are menopausal or not. Because depression is not uncommon, you may develop a depression during these years that is not related to menopause. In addition, since many cases of depression are neither recognized nor treated, you may discover that you are already suffering from an undiagnosed depression.

This chapter will explore

- The symptoms and causes of depression

- The relationship of menopause to depression

- The treatment of depression

- Skills you can use to improve your mood, either in conjunction with professional intervention or by themselves

What Is Depression?

The word depression can be used to describe either a mood or a syndrome. When it is used to describe a mood, it means a feeling of sadness that lasts for a time. Everyone goes through periods of normal sadness, grief over losses, and distress about upsetting situations. Everyone becomes irritable at times and may suffer from some of the symptoms of depression. However, this does not indicate a serious depression. When the word "depression" is used to describe a syndrome, a depressed mood is only one in a whole constellation of symptoms.

When there is a pattern of these symptoms, it is called a syndrome. The importance of a serious depression, or "clinical depression," is that it is thought to be biologically based and to run in families. An untreated depression can cause serious complications, including disruptions in family relationships, problems on the job, and even suicide.

Serious depression affects women at a rate two to three times that of men. A woman's lifetime risk for developing a serious depression ranges from 10 to 25 percent, compared to 5 to 12 percent for men. Rates of depression for women (and men) are highest between the ages of twenty-five and forty-four. In the United States, depression is estimated to cost approximately $44 billion yearly in treatment, absenteeism, and reduced productivity in the workplace.

Symptoms

The symptoms of a serious clinical depression involve noticeable changes from your usual functioning that have lasted for at least two weeks. Use the following checklist to help determine whether you may be suffering from a depressive episode.

Depression Checklist

1. ____ Depressed mood most of the day, nearly every day

2. ____ Significant loss of interest or pleasure in all, or almost all, activities most of the day, nearly every day

3. ____ Significant weight loss (when not dieting) or weight gain

4. ____ Too little or too much sleep nearly every day

5. ____ Noticeable slowing or restlessness nearly every day

6. ____ Fatigue or loss of energy nearly every day

7. ____ Feelings of worthlessness, or excessive or inappropriate guilt nearly every day

8. ____ Difficulty thinking, concentrating, or making decisions nearly every day

9. ____ Recurrent thoughts of death (not just fear of dying), recurrent suicidal ideas without a specific plan, or a suicide attempt or specific plan

If you checked *either* item "1" or "2," *and* at least five symptoms altogether (including "1" and/or "2"), you may be suffering from a serious depression and should seek professional help.

Reprinted with permission from the Diagnostic and Statistical Manual of Mental Disorders, Fourth Edition. Copyright 1994 American Psychiatric Association.

Causes of Serious Depression

Depression is caused by several factors. Recent research has focused on biological and biochemical factors. Many studies suggest some genetic basis for depression because the risk of becoming depressed approximately doubles when an immediate family member has been depressed. There also appears to be an increased risk if a family member is or was an alcoholic or a substance abuser. It is hypothesized that many people who are depressed "self-medicate" with alcohol or drugs to try to alleviate their symptoms. There is also a close association of depression with gender; women suffer from depression twice as often as men. Recent research has shown that the sex hormones may differentially influence brain development in men and women. This influence may increase the vulnerability of women to mood disorders.

In addition to differences related to gender, neurological research has shown that the physical and psychological changes in depression may be related to changes in the availability of certain neurotransmitters, the chemicals that carry signals between the nerve cells in the brain. Neurotransmitters presently implicated in depression include serotonin, norepinephrine, and dopamine. Estrogen also plays a role in neurotransmitter function and enhances mood by altering neurotransmitter activity.

Psychological, cognitive, and social factors may also play a role. Major life changes including death of a loved one, divorce, and illness can trigger a depressive episode. Negative and distorted thinking are frequently seen during depressive episodes, although it is hard to know whether negative thinking causes depression or depression causes negative thinking. Social factors such as poverty, powerlessness, and lack of social support may also be associated with an increased risk of depression.

Depression and Menopause

Research studies have found no increase in the incidence of serious clinical depression in women around the time of menopause when compared with other periods of the female life cycle.

Although there is no increase in depressive episodes, the World Health Organization has found that there is an increase in psychological symptoms in the two years prior to the end of menstrual periods, and a decrease in symptoms in the two years following the last period. The symptoms that were most often experienced were

- Depressed mood
- Loss of confidence
- Forgetfulness
- Fatigue

- Difficulty making decisions
- Anxiety
- Difficulty concentrating
- Feelings of worthlessness

Some of these symptoms, such as fatigue and difficulty in making decisions, while possibly indicitive of depression, may also be due to the sleeplessness associated with hot flashes and night sweats.

However, depression is not uncommon, and if you experience these symptoms it is important to have them evaluated.

Menopause and Women Who Have a History of Depression

There is now a body of evidence that suggests that some women may be at risk for depression associated with menstruation, birth, and menopause. If you have had severe PMS or a postpartum depression, you may become depressed at menopause. If you have had a history of a bipolar disorder (manic-depressive illness), your emotional cycles may change with menopause.

Treatment of Depression

Research has shown both medication and psychotherapy to be effective treatments for serious depressions.

Medical Evaluation and Treatment

If you are being evaluated for depression, you may undergo a complete physical examination to rule out any possible physical causes for depressive symptoms. There are a number of physical conditions that can cause symptoms of depression, such as an underactive thyroid. There are also a number of medications that can cause depressive symptoms, such as some medications for high blood pressure and heart disease (for example, Aldomet and Inderal). Provera can also cause depression.

For mood changes associated with menopause, often the addition of or modification to HRT can alleviate some symptoms (see chapter 6). For example, if HRT allows you to sleep with fewer disturbances from night sweats, you are likely to experience greater concentration, less irritability, and increased levels of energy.

There is some evidence that the level of the neurotransmitter serotonin, (which is felt to be necessary for normal mood) may be lower in the perimenopausal and menopausal years. If your symptoms are suggestive of depression (even if they don't meet the criteria on page 89) and HRT has not been effective in treating it, you may want to consult a physician about the use of antidepressants.

Antidepressants

If your physician determines that antidepressant medication is likely to be helpful to you, it is important to have a basic understanding of this type of treatment. Many different

Table 10.1
Table of Antidepressants

Antidepressant Class	Indications/ Contraindications	Side Effects
Tricyclics (TCAs) Desipramine (Norpramin) Nortriptyline (Pamelor) Imipramine (Trofranil) Amitriptyline (Elavil) Protriptyline (Vivactil) Doxepin (Sinequan)	Due to their sedating effects, TCAs are useful for patients with insomnia. They may pose a risk for individuals with cardiovascular disease, such as arrhythmias.	Most common: dry mouth, constipation. Others: weight gain, dizziness caused by a drop in blood pressure on sitting or standing up (orthostatic hypotension), changes in sexual desire, difficulty urinating, increased sweating, and sedation. TCAs can be lethal in overdose.
Selective Serotonin Reuptake Inhibitors (SSRIs) Fluoxetine (Prozac) Sertraline (Zoloft) Paroxetine (Paxil) Fluvoxamine (Luvox)	SSRIs are generally the first line choice because they have fewer side effects than other antidepressants, do not require blood monitoring, and are safe in overdose.	Insomnia, agitation, sexual dysfunction, occasional nausea or heartburn, headache, occasional drowsiness, dizziness, tremor, diarrhea/constipation, and dry mouth (rare).
Monoamine Oxidase Inhibitors (MAOIs) Isocarboxazid (Marplan) Tranylcypromine (Parnate) Phenelzine (Nardil)	Can cause severe and sudden rise in blood pressure if ingested with certain drugs (e.g., over-the-counter cold preparations, diet pills, and amphetamines), or foods containing tyramine, (e.g., red wines, aged cheeses). Interact with epinephrine in some topical anesthetics. Not advised with other antidepressants.	Agitation, insomnia, sexual dysfunction, disturbed appetite, faintness (like orthostatic hypotension). Weight gain is most prominent with MAOIs.
Bupropion (Wellbutrin)	Doesn't interact significantly with other drugs. At high doses can cause seizures in some people, most commonly those who have seizure disorders, anorexia, or bulima. Used experimentally to counteract sexual side effects of SSRIs.	Agitation, insomnia, sedation, blurred vision, dizziness, headache/migraine, dry mouth, tremor, appetite loss, weight loss, excessive sweating, rapid heart beats, constipation, rashes.
Trazodone (Desyrel)	Often used with another antidepressant to alleviate insomnia induced by the initial drug.	Drowsiness, faintness, nausea, and vomiting.

Antidepressant Class	Indications/ Contraindications	Side Effects
Maprotiline (Ludiomil)	To treat agitation and anxiety associated with depression. Not advised for people with seizure disorders. Somewhat risky for patients with cardiovascular disease.	Adverse reactions are similar to TCAs.
Serotonin and Norepinephrine Reuptake Inhibitors (SNRIs) Venlafaxine (Effexor)	Works something like a combination of an SSRI and a tricyclic might. Useful for patients who don't respond to other antidepressants.	Similar to those of SSRIs.
Nefazodone (Serzone)	Shouldn't be taken with the non-sedating antihist-amines, terfenadine (Seldane) and astemizone (Hismanal).	Headache, dry mouth, nausea, drowsiness, faintness, constipation.

Source: *Harvard Women's Health Watch*, December 1995.

types of antidepressant medication exist (see table 10.1). It is thought that all antidepressants work by increasing the effectiveness of several neurotransmitters in the brain. Although all antidepressants can be effective, they may take from four to eight weeks at a therapeutic dosage to work. Many people stop treatment prematurely because they do not get an immediate response. That is why it is important to work closely with your physician.

All antidepressants can have side effects. Side effects are still the most common reason for switching from one drug to another. It is impossible to know in advance what side effects you might have, so a trial of more than one medication may be required if side effects are intolerable.

Antidepressants are not addicting. They should be taken exactly as prescribed. You will probably need to remain on medication after your symptoms are completely gone for at least ten to twelve months. If you have had multiple episodes of depression, longer term therapy may be necessary.

As with any prescription medication, antidepressants must be prescribed and moni-tored by a competent physician who is familiar with their use. Although some primary care physicians do prescribe antidepressants, psychiatrists are the physicians who specialize in and are most familiar with these medications.

Estrogen. In nondepressed women, estrogen enhances mood; so when its level diminishes, there can be a decline of mood in many women. If you experience a first episode of a mild-to-moderate depression during perimenopause, an appropriate treatment strategy is to use estrogen to alleviate symptoms of short-lasting mood swings, irritability, feelings

---

What to Ask Your Doctor About Medication

- What are the possible side effects and risks?

- How long will it be before the medication begins to help?

- Do I have to eat or avoid eating when I take this medicine?

- Will it affect my ability to work, drive, or operate machinery?

- Should I call you if any particular side effects develop?

- Is there any danger from skipping a dose? From taking a double dose?

- Does this medicine interact with any other medications, including over-the-counter medicines?

- Are there any foods or substances, such as alcohol, that I should avoid?

- How long will I have to take this medication?

- What are the alternatives to using this drug?

- What if this drug doesn't work?

Source: *Caring for the Mind,* Diane Hales and Robert E. Hales, M.D. Copyright 1995 by Dianne Hales and Robert E. Hales, M.D. Used by permission of Bantam Books, a division of Bantam Doubleday Dell Publishing Group, Inc.

of sadness, and crying spells. For severe depression, antidepressants are the treatment of choice. Estrogen may increase the effect of antidepressants and may therefore allow a reduction in their dosage. Research has not yet determined the value of adding estrogen to women with a chronic long-standing depression who are not responding to antidepressants and psychotherapy.

If estrogen is used, progestin should be added to protect the uterus against endometrial hyperplasia. However, since many women have mood changes with progestin, the lowest dose required to prevent endometrial hyperplasia is recommended.

Whenever you are prescribed a new medication for any condition, it is important to take charge and be knowledgeable about what you are taking. Refer to the box for questions you might want to ask your physician about the medication.

Psychotherapy

There are many psychological therapies that can be used to treat depression:

IPT, or interpersonal psychotherapy, is a brief (twelve to sixteen week) treatment. Since depression occurs in an interpersonal context, interventions are directed at this interpersonal context. Four problem areas are focused on: grief, conflict with others, role transitions, and interpersonal deficits. A clear treatment strategy is then developed for each problem area.

Cognitive therapy, also a brief therapy, focuses on the connection between negative thinking and depression. After identifying thinking distortions and inaccurate beliefs, you learn to change those negative thought patterns to more constructive ones. An improvement in mood follows the improvement in thinking.

Psychodynamic psychotherapy looks at conscious and unconscious issues underlying your present problems and concerns, and takes developmental issues into consideration.

Supportive psychotherapy offers a safe, therapeutic environment where the therapist provides an atmosphere to listen and validate your feelings. This process will help you clarify your thoughts, feelings, and options.

All methods can be effective if utilized by someone who is an expert in that particular form of therapy.

What to expect from therapy

Psychotherapy is provided by a number of different mental health professionals, including psychiatrists, psychologists, social workers, marriage and family counselors, and psychiatric nurses. However, only psychiatrists can assess the contribution of biology and are able to prescribe medication if indicated. If you are treated with both medication and psychotherapy, you may be working with two different mental health professionals simultaneously—a psychiatrist who will evaluate, prescribe, and monitor your medication, and a psychotherapist for the psychotherapy or counseling.

Over the first few visits, the mental health professional should take a history to find out about your current psychological problem, past emotional problems, and a family history of mental illness or substance abuse. In addition, a medical history, a list of the medications that you are currently taking, and whether you are currently using or have a history of using drugs and alcohol are useful in determining if you may need further medical evaluation.

During the first few visits, you may develop a set of goals and a treatment plan. For example, the goal may be to resolve a specific crisis, or you may want to be treated for general depression. If your benefits are limited by managed care or your insurance plan, your goals may be tailored to what can be reasonably accomplished within those limits.

Because psychotherapy uses the patient/therapist relationship to effect change, it is important that you feel comfortable with your therapist. This does not mean that there will not be times when you might feel uncomfortable as new issues emerge, but you should have a sense of trust that your therapist has your best interest in mind so you can freely express your feelings. Therapy is an active process. It is not passive. Your therapist will be asking you questions, making comments, and even offering suggestions to help you move in the most productive direction.

Therapists often use their own emotional responses during the session as a guide to understanding your interpersonal issues and style. If you are uncomfortable with anything the therapist does or says, you are encouraged to discuss it. Remember that your therapist should never behave in a way that makes you sexually uncomfortable. If this is the case, it is important to seek a second opinion.

If after a few sessions you feel that you have not made progress in therapy, you are encouraged to discuss this concern. If the discussion does not yield positive results, you might consider changing to another therapist.

Other Activities to Improve Mood

Other activities can be very helpful in alleviating depressive symptoms, either with professional treatment or by themselves. For example, support groups can be excellent sources of education, social support, and brainstorming. They can also reduce feelings of isolation and stigma. (See chapter 15 for more information on support groups.) Self-help books, like this one, can also be beneficial. You will find a list of recommended books for depression in appendix E.

Do Something

Research has shown that "doing something is better than doing nothing." Just about any activity is helpful, but pleasurable activities are especially helpful in elevating your mood. Many people, when they're feeling depressed, say, "Oh, I'll do it later, when I'm feeling better. I don't feel like doing that right now." The paradox is that "doing something" is one of the best ways to make yourself feel better! Use the following suggestions to increase your activities. Look at the sample chart before you try it on your own. Feel free to photocopy the blank chart for your continued use.

Increasing Activity in Your Life

- Create a schedule for yourself, making sure that you include pleasurable activities. You can also use pleasurable activities as a reward for having worked on unpleasurable activities.

- If you write your schedule down, you're more likely to do it.

- Include companions in your activities, because once you've made a commitment to someone else, you are more likely to do it.

- Make sure your schedule is realistic, and remember that even if you don't feel like doing something or going somewhere, as soon as you start, you'll probably begin to feel better almost immediately.

- Make a deal with yourself that you'll try something for 20 minutes with an open attitude. If you're objectively not feeling any better after the 20 minutes, you can stop.

Sample Activity Schedule
Day: Saturday

Time	Activity	Companion	Reward	Check if Done
8:30 AM	Write bills	No one	Read newspaper	✔
10:00 AM	Swim	Sarah	None necessary—I know I'll feel better	✔
Noon	Housework for 45 minutes	No one	Read novel for an hour	✔
3:00 PM	Grocery shop	No one	Buy my favorite exotic fruit	✔
5:00 PM	Phone Vicki	Vicki	This is a reward	✔
6:30 PM	Dinner with Bill	Bill	Another reward	✔

Exercise

Exercise has already been discussed in the context of osteoporosis and lifestyle changes, and will be discussed later in regard to stress management. Exercise also helps your mood. Many antidepressants increase the amount of serotonin available in the brain. When you exercise, (especially when you exercise vigorously) short-term changes in brain chemistry occur that promote feelings of well-being and an improvement in mood. You are urged to exercise daily if your physician concurs, as well as any time you are experiencing distressing emotions. Look at chapter 8 for additional information and suggestions for developing and maintaining a lifelong exercise program.

Activity Schedule
Day:_____

Time	Activity	Companion	Reward	Check if Done

Support

Support from friends and family members is essential to maintain optimal moods. Yet when you're feeling depressed, you often don't feel that you're "fit company" for others, or are afraid you'll "bring them down" or alienate them. Let others know if you're feeling sad, and let them know what they can or can't do for you. If you tell someone that you don't need them to make you feel better or take away your bad mood, but you just want them to listen, they'll know what to do and won't feel powerless or frustrated. If you want someone to join you in an activity, and you clarify your wish, that, too, will steer them in the right direction, and will optimize the likelihood that you'll get what you need. Look at chapter 13 for additional tips on communication.

People show their support and caring in different ways. Some, for example, will be good listeners, while others will offer to do things for you. Unless you know how someone else shows their support, you may miss their efforts. Alternatively, as mentioned above, you can ask people to provide you with specific kinds of support, so that you're both in agreement.

The chart on the following page will help you identify who is supportive in your life, in what ways, and how supportive they are. Once you are more clear on who in your life is most capable of supporting you in certain ways, you can identify what you need, and ask the person most likely to be able to provide it. This should optimize your chances of getting your needs met.

Summary

- There is a difference between depression as a mood and serious depression as a syndrome.

- Serious depression is the most common emotional problem in women.

- Evaluation and treatment of serious depression is very important.

- Both medication and psychotherapy can be extremely helpful.

- Other pursuits, such as exercise, social support, and increased activity can make a big difference in your mood, whether or not you're clinically depressed.

Who Are the Supportive People in Your Life?

Relationship	Name	Types of Support	Level (1–5) *with higher scores indicating more support*
Sample: Partner	JOHN	Giving me ideas	5
		Listening	3
Partner			
Family members			
Friends			
Others			

11

Maximize Your Mood

Whether or not you suffer from a mood disorder, you can benefit greatly from some mood-maximizing skills borrowed from cognitive therapy. Often a low mood is associated with negative thinking. This chapter will explore

- How to identify negative thinking patterns

- How to change your thinking to improve your mood

These techniques are not meant as a substitute for psychotherapy. However, they can be useful in conjunction with psychotherapy or as a strategy you can use on your own to feel better.

Cognitive therapy emphasizes the identification and modification of distorted thinking styles. Thinking is one word used to describe the ongoing internal conversation you have with yourself every waking moment. Another term to describe this process is *self-talk*. Over the years, most people have developed some bad habits with regard to self-talk. Your mood will improve when your self-talk is more positive.

Several authors have written extensively about distorted thinking, which is associated with depressed moods. Many forms of cognitive distortions have been identified. The following list includes some of the most common forms. See how many of these styles you can identify in your own thinking.

Common Styles of Distorted Thinking

Place a check next to each style that applies to your self-talk.

1. _____ **Filtering.** You focus on one negative aspect of a situation to the exclusion of everything else, and you allow this detail to color the entire event. It is often accompanied by words such as "terrible," "awful," or "horrible." Example: "Whenever my brother calls, my day is ruined."

2. _____ **Black-or-white thinking.** You tend to see everything as an extreme, with very little room for a middle ground. Anything short of excellence is a failure. Example: The person who has a cigarette after she's stopped smoking, and says, "Oh, now I've blown it."

3. _____ **Global labeling.** Taking black-or-white thinking to even greater extremes, you focus on only one aspect or quality in yourself, a situation, or other people, and apply a negative label to it. Example: Your coworker who refused to give you a lift home is a total jerk.

4. _____ **Overgeneralization.** In this distortion, you reach very broad conclusions based on a single incident or piece of evidence. It is often accompanied by absolute words, such as *always*, *never*, *nobody*, or *everyone*. Examples: "Nobody loves me." "I could never get a better job." "No one would stay my friend if they really knew me."

5. _____ **Mind reading.** You make negative assumptions about other people without any information to support your conclusions. Example: You assume that someone who is not paying attention to you during a conversation finds you boring or dumb, rather than thinking that they might be preoccupied that day.

6. _____ **Crystal ball gazing.** This distortion is similar to mind reading, but relates to negative assumptions about the future. At its worst, crystal ball gazing becomes catastrophizing, in which you predict the worst-case scenario. Examples: A headache leads you to believe you have a brain tumor. You assume that you won't do well at an interview, or that you won't get a promotion.

7. _____ **Personalization.** This is the tendency to relate everything that occurs around you to yourself, often comparing yourself to others or blaming yourself for an outcome. Example: A man whose wife complains about rising prices hears the complaints as attacks on his abilities as a breadwinner.

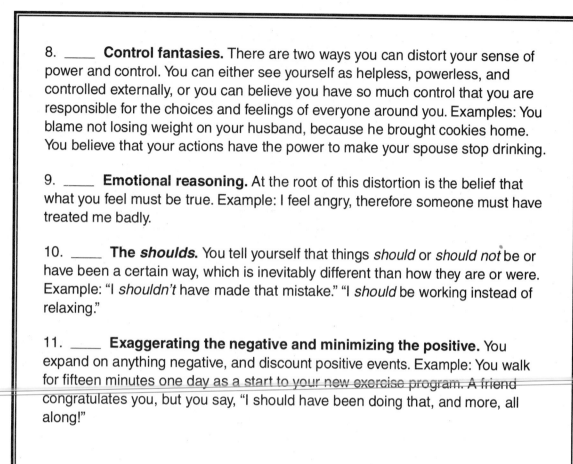

8. ____ **Control fantasies.** There are two ways you can distort your sense of power and control. You can either see yourself as helpless, powerless, and controlled externally, or you can believe you have so much control that you are responsible for the choices and feelings of everyone around you. Examples: You blame not losing weight on your husband, because he brought cookies home. You believe that your actions have the power to make your spouse stop drinking.

9. ____ **Emotional reasoning.** At the root of this distortion is the belief that what you feel must be true. Example: I feel angry, therefore someone must have treated me badly.

10. ____ **The *shoulds*.** You tell yourself that things *should* or *should not* be or have been a certain way, which is inevitably different than how they are or were. Example: "I *shouldn't* have made that mistake." "I *should* be working instead of relaxing."

11. ____ **Exaggerating the negative and minimizing the positive.** You expand on anything negative, and discount positive events. Example: You walk for fifteen minutes one day as a start to your new exercise program. A friend congratulates you, but you say, "I should have been doing that, and more, all along!"

If you're like most people, you can identify with many of these destructive forms of self-talk and have made several check marks. However, labeling yourself negatively for using them, or telling yourself that you shouldn't use them anymore, won't help the problem. It will be more constructive to learn to change these negative thinking habits by replacing them with new, constructive thinking habits.

The only way to develop a new habit is to practice the behavior enough so that it becomes a habit. That requires developing a higher level of awareness of your self-talk, so that you can short-circuit your "automatic pilot" and make a conscious, positive choice about how you talk to yourself. To accomplish this goal, practice with the following Five Column Technique. Whenever you feel distressed, depressed, angry, or frustrated, or you experience some other significant negative emotion, take a "time-out" and use this technique. It will help you minimize the negative emotion. However, the technique will be most helpful if you've practiced it beforehand. Read the directions and look at the sample first, then try it on your own.

Five Column Technique

Directions: To use this technique, think of one or two events in the recent past in which you have experienced distressing emotions. Try to remember exactly what you said to yourself about the situation, word for word. You'll record these thoughts in column 1 (Initial Self-Talk).

Then recall the emotions that you experienced—the emotions that your thoughts about the situation evoked. Record those in column 2 (Emotional Reaction).

Now, return to the "Common Styles of Distorted Thinking" list and try to pick out the types you used in your self-talk. Some of the forms are similar, so you might find that you've used three or four (or more) different types. Record these in column 3 (Dysfunctional Thought Patterns).

The next step is to try to come up with some rational, constructive responses to your thoughts. For help with this, look at the list on page 107, "Combatting Your Distortions." Just brainstorm here; no one is going to grade you. You can even ask supportive friends and family members for help—you'll be teaching them about constructive thinking at the same time as helping yourself. Record these constructive thoughts in column 4 (Restructured Thoughts).

Finally, become aware of any changes in your emotional reactions (hopefully positive!), and record these in column 5 (New Emotional Reaction).

Here's an example:

Event: You've begun a weight control program. You've been doing really well, eating lots of fruit and vegetables, staying away from red meat, lowering the fat content of your food, drinking lots of water, and walking. You've lost five pounds already. However, someone brings fresh, homemade, chocolate chip cookies into the office, which just happens to be your favorite food of all time. You eat two cookies.

Initial Self-Talk	Emotional Reaction	Dysfunctional Thought Patterns	Restructured Thoughts	New Emotional Reaction
"You're an idiot! Why did you do that? Now you've blown it. You'll never lose weight. You have no willpower. What's wrong with you, anyway? I can't believe you did that!"	Guilt, disgust, anger at myself	Global labeling ("You're an idiot!") Black-or-white thinking ("Now you've blown it.") Over-generalization Crystal Ball Gazing ("You'll never lose weight.")	"Well, it's certainly not the end of the world. Two chocolate chip cookies are only about 200 calories; that's about 1/18th of a pound. You've been doing really well, and you know the thing that will make you feel best is to get right back on track. You don't have to wait until tomorrow. Eat your regular lunch, so you won't get too hungry in the afternoon, and maybe you can take an extra walk this week."	I feel much better about myself and optimistic again about my health plan.

Now, try it on your own. Remember to refer to the lists.

Event: _____

_____

_____

_____

Initial Self-Talk	Emotional Reaction	Dysfunctional Thought Patterns	Restructured Thoughts	New Emotional Reaction

As you're doing these exercises, remember that your goal is not to rid yourself entirely of *every* feeling. Feelings are useful. They can give you significant information about yourself and your environment. However, when your feelings are based on irrational beliefs and interpretations about your environment, you can make yourself feel much better by separating out the irrational parts, so that you can see the situations more clearly and objectively.

It is also important to recognize that you will not change overnight. After all, you have probably gotten pretty good at any habit you've practiced for thirty or forty years. Even if you change very slowly, with a lot of slips, you will be moving in the right direction. Even if you don't catch yourself until the next day, you're learning. You'll find that the "time lag" becomes shorter with practice, until there will be many times where you'll catch yourself while you're distorting your thinking. With enough practice, you'll be able to anticipate and catch yourself beforehand much of the time.

Combatting Your Distortions

1. **Filtering.** Identify key words and replace them with more constructive alternatives. For example:

Key words:	Alternatives:
terrible	unexpected
horrible	unplanned
awful	unpleasant

2. **Black-or-white thinking.** Think about things in percentages from 0 to 100 (and you can't use "0" or "100"). For example, "I was 40 percent successful in sticking to my food plan today."

3. **Global labeling.** Try to focus on the big picture rather than only a single characteristic. Ask yourself if the label is always accurate, only accurate now, or only accurate some of the time. Also, rather than apply a negative label to yourself, identify what you can learn from a situation and how you might be able to apply it in the future. This approach works well for black-or-white thinking, also.

4. **Overgeneralization.** The key word method can also be helpful. For example:

Key words:	Alternatives:
always, never	sometimes, occasionally
no one, everyone	some people

5. **Mind reading, crystal ball gazing, and personalization.** It is helpful to treat all of your assumptions about people and situations as guesses. For mind reading and personalization, you might check out the guesses by asking the person in question or examining the evidence. For crystal ball gazing, make an honest assessment of the situation in terms of odds. For example, "Realistically, the probability that I have a brain tumor is close to zero."

6. **Control fantasies.** Honesty is also the key. Try to accept the responsibility for your choices, without negatively judging yourself, and try to allow others to accept the responsibility for their choices.

7. **Emotional reasoning.** Rather than believing that reality is dependent on how you feel, try to remember that what you *feel* is often dependent on what you *think*, and your *thinking* may be distorted.

8. **The *shoulds*.** It's important to realize that there are exceptions to almost every rule. Try to find exceptions to the rule you've created with your *should*. The key word system also works well here. The key words include *should, shouldn't, ought, must*. Replace them with statements like "I wish I hadn't made that mistake," or "I'd like to exercise today."

9. **Exaggerating the negative and minimizing the positive.** Try to turn it around by focusing only on the positive. For example, "Good for me, fifteen minutes of walking is a lot better than no minutes!"

Summary

- Distortions caused by negative thinking are associated with depressed moods.

- There are common forms of distorted thinking that you can identify.

- Once identified, you can combat your distortions.

- As your thinking becomes more positive, your mood will improve.

12

Manage Your Stress Before It
Manages You!

Stress is a fact of life and, like it or not, we have to deal with it. Each stage of life has its own unique challenges, and while it is important not to exaggerate the stresses of midlife, it is also important not to make the opposite mistake and minimize them. Some women are fearful of communicating their stress because they believe their significant others will say, "Oh, it's all in your head," or "What do you expect? You're just going through 'the change.'"

While having too much stress in your life can certainly be debilitating, it can also give you the motivation and opportunity to change your life in healthy ways. This chapter will

- Help you clarify the meaning of the word *stress*

- Explore the causes and consequences of stress

- Help you design an individualized stress management plan

Causes and Consequences of Stress

It will be helpful to begin by defining *stress*. Although we all talk about stress freely in daily conversation, the word is often misunderstood. Stress refers to a complex physical response in our bodies that occurs every time our environment changes. This response, called the *stress response*, can probably be traced back to prehistoric times, when it served to help our species survive: A cavewoman stepped out of her cave, only to come face-to-face (or face-to-fang) with a threatening animal. A chain reaction in her body occurred, preparing her for a *fight-or-flight* response. The blood rushed to her muscles, her heart rate sped up, and other bodily changes occurred, readying her to either fight the animal or to run away. While following either one of those courses of action, the cavewoman used up her excess physical energy, and was able to relax after it was over.

That worked well for the cavewoman, however, for you it's a little different. When you're stuck in freeway traffic, you can't very well fight (ram into the car in front of you) or flee (leave the scene). When your boss gives you a stressful assignment, you can't very well fight (beat up the boss) or flee (leave work). The consequence is that you're not allowed to complete the stress response and return to a natural, relaxed state. Your excess physical (nervous) energy has nowhere to go, and you're left feeling the consequences of unrelieved stress.

Stress, then, is any change requiring adaptation. A more common way of thinking about it, and a practical definition for this chapter is as follows: *Stress is the reaction that occurs when the demands placed upon us exceed our resources.* Most of us think that only negative changes cause stress. However, any change, even a positive change, can be stressful until you have adapted to it. When you think about it, positive events like your child's marriage, vacations, and holidays can be very stressful.

To learn more about your sources of stress, look at the "Change Checklist" on the following page. It is a list of life changes, all of which can be stressful. Place a check mark beside those that you have experienced within the past year.

There is an association between stressful life experiences and illness. Although there is still a lot that is not understood about this association, if you have recently experienced poor health, you may find the following exercise to be of special interest. Look at the checklist on page 112 of symptoms of stress, and place a check mark beside those that you've experienced lately. While it is important to have any physical symptoms reviewed by your physician, if he or she is unable to find a physical cause for them, they may be stress related. Total the number of symptoms you checked, and use the following scale to determine your stress level.

0–5	You're doing great!
5–8	**Mild to Moderate Stress Level.** You show some signs of stress and are likely to find the information in this chapter useful to ease your stress.
9–16	**Moderate to Severe Stress Level.** Stress is having a significant impact on your life. Professional help should be considered.
17+	**Severe Stress Level.** You are strongly encouraged to seek a professional's evaluation and counseling to reduce your stress level.

Change Checklist

Personal

- [ ] Aging
- [ ] Buying/selling a car
- [ ] Change in emotional outlook
- [ ] Change in financial status
- [ ] Change in habit
  - [ ] alcohol
  - [ ] drugs
  - [ ] tobacco
  - [ ] exercise
  - [ ] nutrition
- [ ] Change in religious views/beliefs
- [ ] Change in roles
- [ ] Change in self-concept
- [ ] Personal injury/illness handicap
- [ ] Other: _____

Work

- [ ] Change in hours
- [ ] Change in job security
- [ ] Change in relationships at work
- [ ] Change in workload
- [ ] Change in pay
- [ ] Promotion/demotion
- [ ] Retirement
- [ ] Starting new job
- [ ] Strike
- [ ] Other: _____

Family

- [ ] Change in recreation patterns
- [ ] Death of close friend(s) or family member(s)
- [ ] Family member(s) leaving home
- [ ] Illness/healing of family member(s)
- [ ] Marriage
- [ ] New family member(s)
- [ ] Parent/child tensions
- [ ] Partner stopping or starting a job
- [ ] Separation/divorce
- [ ] Trouble with in-laws
- [ ] Other: _____

Environment

- [ ] Crime against property
- [ ] Holiday(s)
- [ ] Major house cleaning
- [ ] Moving to new
  - [ ] City
  - [ ] Climate
  - [ ] Culture
  - [ ] House or apartment
  - [ ] Neighborhood
- [ ] Natural disaster
- [ ] Remodeling
- [ ] Vacation
- [ ] War
- [ ] Other: _____

Reprinted with permission from *Structured Exercises in Stress Management, Volume 1,* copyright 1983, 1994. Donald A. Tubesing. Published by Whole Person Associates Inc, 210 West Michigan, Duluth, MN 55802-1908

Stress Symptoms

Emotional

- ☐ Anxiety
- ☐ Bad temper
- ☐ Crying spells
- ☐ Depression
- ☐ Easily discouraged
- ☐ Frustration
- ☐ Irritability
- ☐ Little joy
- ☐ Mood swings
- ☐ Nervous laugh
- ☐ Nightmares
- ☐ "No one cares"
- ☐ The "blues"
- ☐ Worrying

Mental

- ☐ Boredom
- ☐ Confusion
- ☐ Dull senses
- ☐ Forgetfulness
- ☐ Indifference
- ☐ Low productivity
- ☐ Negative attitude
- ☐ Negative self-talk
- ☐ No new ideas
- ☐ Poor concentration
- ☐ Spacing out
- ☐ Whirling mind
- ☐ Unnecessary risk taking

Physical

- ☐ Accident prone
- ☐ Appetite change
- ☐ Colds
- ☐ Fatigue
- ☐ Finger drumming
- ☐ Foot tapping
- ☐ Headaches
- ☐ Increased alcohol, drug, tobacco use
- ☐ Insomnia
- ☐ Lethargy
- ☐ Muscle aches
- ☐ Pounding heart
- ☐ Rash
- ☐ Restlessness
- ☐ Teeth grinding
- ☐ Tension
- ☐ Weight change

Relational

- ☐ Clamming up
- ☐ Distrust
- ☐ Fewer contacts with friends
- ☐ Hiding
- ☐ Intolerance
- ☐ Isolation
- ☐ Lack of intimacy
- ☐ Lashing out
- ☐ Loneliness
- ☐ Lowered sex drive
- ☐ Nagging
- ☐ Resentment
- ☐ Using people

Spiritual

- ☐ Apathy
- ☐ Cynicism
- ☐ Doubt
- ☐ Emptiness
- ☐ Looking for magic
- ☐ Loss of direction
- ☐ Loss of meaning
- ☐ Martyrdom
- ☐ Needing to "prove" self
- ☐ Unforgiving

Reprinted with permission from *Structured Exercises in Stress Management, Volume 1*, copyright 1983, 1994. Donald A. Tubesing. Published by Whole Person Associates Inc, 210 West Michigan, Duluth, MN 55802-1908

You can't stop changes from occurring in your life. Even if you could, you would not want to stop them, because, surprisingly, too little stress can have its own problems. There is a relationship between stress and productivity, and it looks something like this:

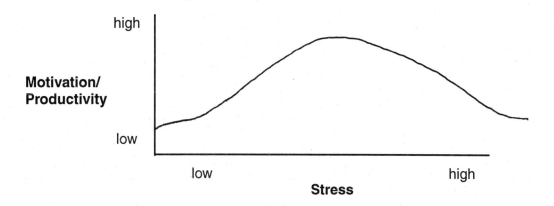

Although you often talk about wanting a stress-free life, if you got rid of all stress, you would have little motivation to do the things that give you enjoyment and provide meaning in life. However, when your stress level is too high, you become paralyzed and lose productivity. A manageable level of stress is acceptable and can be challenging as long as it is not overwhelming.

Managing Your Stress

If you have too much stress in your life, what can you do about it? The rest of this chapter provides a comprehensive approach for managing stress more effectively. As you read this, you will find it helpful to identify one currently stressful situation in your life so you can practice using the techniques.

There are three important steps to managing stress:

Step 1: Change the situation.

Step 2: Change your reaction to the situation.

Step 3: Increase your tolerance of and preparedness for stress.

The first two steps address changing things you *can* change, while the third is about becoming better able to accept those things you *can't* change.

Step 1: Change the situation.

When you approach a problematic and stressful situation in your life, it's easy to feel overwhelmed and become mentally paralyzed. In order to prevent that, keep in mind the following maxim:

Although you may not be able to entirely solve a problem, you can, in most cases, solve some part(s) of it. Eventually, the small dents can make a large impact.

Remember that any choices you make are likely to have both positive and negative consequences. As human beings, you often suffer the misconception that if you think long and hard enough, you will be able to come up with the "right" or "perfect solution." Unfortunately, such a solution rarely exists.

The next time you make a decision, you may experience some inevitable negative consequences. Try to keep the following in mind as you cope with those consequences:

- Remember that another choice may just as easily have resulted in an equal number of both positive and negative consequences.

- As soon as you reduce the need to try to please everyone, you can make decisions more easily.

- Recognize the impossibility of pleasing everyone at the same time.

- Acknowledge that you're trying to make the most thoughtful and best decision you can.

- Define the problem accurately.

Accurate problem definition may be the most important and difficult aspect of problem solving. When you accurately and specifically define a problem, you may learn that, in actuality, it's not your problem. Sometimes you think you have a problem, when you don't have the responsibility or the control that would be required to solve it. In those cases, you need to work on gradually and gently letting go. Remember, your control only extends as far as your fingertips (and sometimes not even that far!).

On the next page is a guide that can be helpful in your problem-solving ventures. First, there is a sample guide. Then, a blank guide is provided for you to photocopy and use whenever it's necessary.

Step 2: Change your reaction to situations.

So far, you've seen how you can make changes in the problem areas of your life in order to reduce stress. The next step does not involve changing the situation, but rather aims to reduce stress by making changes in your reaction to the situation. You have already learned to do this in chapter 11 when you learned the Five Column Technique to identify and change the unhelpful thinking patterns that cause distressing reactions. In that chapter, you applied

Steps to Problem Solving (Sample)

Here is an example of how you can use this exercise.

A. **Summarize your symptoms.** How do you know there is a problem? What signs are indicating stress in your life? (You can look back at your responses to "Stress Symptoms" for help.)

I'm having trouble sleeping.

I'm worried and angry.

B. **Define the problem from several perspectives.** What is the source of your stress? Write three or four different descriptions of the problem. Indicate which one most clearly captures the cause of your stress.

1. *I believe my mother is living in an unsafe environment. She lives alone, and has fallen and lives in an unsafe neighborhood.*

2. *My mother won't listen to me. She's stubborn and independent.*

3. *I'm anxious and frustrated about a situation I have no control over.*

C. **Learn from your previous attempts to solve the problem.** What strategies have you already tried? Why didn't they work? What new strategies are suggested by these?

I've tried telling her what she should do. She got defensive. I've tried taking her to retirement homes. She got belligerent. Maybe the new strategy should avoid trying to get her to do something she doesn't want to.

D. **Check your attitude.** How hopeful are you about your capacity to deal with this problem?

Hopeless   Doubtful   Maybe   Possible   Hopeful

What about your desire to tackle the problem and do something about it?

Not motivated   Partially committed   Willing to try   Highly motivated

E. **Identify your resources.** What special strengths and skills can you bring to bear on the problem? What about resources (people, organizations) outside of yourself?

My strengths: caring, persistence

Other resources: local university, books, local hospital, counselor

F. **Specify your goals.** What do you want to happen? to feel? to change? to accomplish? to increase or decrease? to learn? How will you know when the problem is solved? Be specific.

I want *to feel less anxious and angry.*

I want *my mother to be safe.*

I want *to learn new ways to approach my mother.*

What would you have to give up in order to reach your goals? Are you willing to make this sacrifice? Are there some aspects of your problem you'd rather not change right now?

Well, I don't want to seriously injure the relationship with my mother by forcing her to do something against her will. But I think, maybe, by using a different approach, I might make a little more headway. I have to keep in mind that I can't control another person, and the need to control is what I have to give up.

G. **Formulate a clear plan of action.** Based on the changes you want to make and the goals you've set, what, specifically, could you do?

I could *change my approach by letting my mother know I can understand her feelings and instead of being forceful, I could ask her if she could help me be less anxious by making some changes.*

I could *ask my mother to come up with some compromises to resolve our conflict. See if there are small changes she'd be willing to make, like having a helper come for one or two hours a day.*

I could *realize that as long as she's cognitively intact, I have no control over this situation and could work on letting go of it.*

I could *do some relaxation exercises and use some techniques in this book to try to change my thinking so I could decrease my worry and anger.*

Now, what exactly will you plan to do? Include details on frequency, starting point, ending point, and so on.

I will *talk to my mother, validate her feelings, and express to her my fears and anxieties. I'll ask her to help me with my problem, and ask her how she could help me.*

I will *spend ten minutes three times each week with my journal, reviewing the limits of my control and recognizing the impossibility of controlling someone else.*

I will *listen to my relaxation tape three times each week.*

I will *review the Five Column Technique in chapter 11 with regard to this problem two times each week for three weeks.*

H. **Reward yourself.** What special treats will you give to yourself when you accomplish each part of your plan?

When I finish *talking to my mother,*

    I will *go out for lunch with a friend rather than eating my boring low-calorie frozen dinner in the office.*

When I finish *my journal, relaxation, or Five Column Technique work,*

    I will *read a novel for thirty minutes without guilt.*

I. **Follow-up.** How is this plan working? Do you need to modify it? If so, how?

Mom did agree to get a security system and have twice daily phone calls. It's not much, but we agreed to review it in two months. I'm feeling less anxious, angry, and frustrated. It's not entirely gone, but it's better.

Steps to Problem Solving

A. **Summarize your Symptoms.** How do you know there is a problem? What signs are indicating stress in your life? (You can look back at your responses to "Stress Symptoms" for help.) _____

_____

B. **Define the Problem from Several Perspectives.** What is the source of your stress? Write three or four different descriptions of the problem. Indicate which one most clearly captures the cause of your stress.

1. _____

_____

2. _____

_____

3. _____

_____

4. _____

_____

C. **Learn from your previous attempts to solve the problem.** What strategies have you already tried? Why didn't they work? What new strategies are suggested by these? _____

_____

D. **Check your attitude.** How hopeful are you about your capacity to deal with this problem?

Hopeless   Doubtful   Maybe   Possible   Hopeful

What about your desire to tackle the problem and do something about it?

Not motivated   Partially committed   Willing to try   Highly motivated

E. **Identify your resources.** What special strengths and skills can you bring to bear on the problem? What about resources (people, organizations, and so on.) outside of yourself? _____

_____

F. **Specify your goals.** What do you want to happen? to feel? to change? to accomplish? to increase or decrease? to learn? How will you know when the problem is solved? Be specific.

I want _____

_____

I want _____

_____

I want _____

_____

I want _____

_____

What would you have to give up in order to reach your goals? Are you willing to make this sacrifice? Are there some aspects of your problem you'd rather not change right now?

_____

_____

_____

G. **Formulate a clear plan of action.** Based on the changes you want to make and the goals you've set, what, specifically, could you do?

I could _____

_____

I could _____

_____

I could _____

_____

I could _____

_____

Now, what exactly will you plan to do? Include details on frequency, starting point, ending point, and so on.

I will _____

_____

I will _____

_____

I will _____

_____

I will _____

_____

H. **Reward yourself.** What special treats will you give to yourself when you accomplish each part of your plan?

When I finish _____

I will _____

When I finish _____

I will _____

When I finish _____

I will _____

When I finish _____

I will _____

I. Follow-up. How is this plan working? Do you need to modify it? If so, how?

_____

_____

_____

_____

_____

_____

_____

_____

Reprinted with permission from *Structured Exercises in Stress Management, Volume 1*, copyright 1983, 1994. Donald A. Tubesing. Published by Whole Person Associates, Inc. 210 West Michigan, Duluth, MN 55802-1908.

the technique to reduce depressive reactions. Now the same technique will be used to reduce stressful reactions. Remember, this step involves understanding that your interpretation of events and how you talk to yourself about them can actually have a greater impact on your emotional reactions than the event itself. If you can learn to change the way you talk to yourself, you can change your emotional reaction and make it less stressful. Now would be a good time to practice the Five Column Technique with the current stressful situation you've identified for this chapter.

While not all the stress was eliminated, it is clear that by using these techniques, you can certainly make a dent in it.

Step 3: Increase your tolerance of and preparedness for stress.

No matter how many strategies you use, there will always be some stress in life. Step 3 is designed to place your body and mind in a state of readiness to respond optimally to these unavoidable stressors, and to increase the ability to endure or adapt to unfavorable situations that are unchangeable.

The purpose of this step is to develop a personal stress management program—a daily plan for small things you can do to better tolerate the unchangeable stress in your life. Don't expect to develop or completely implement this program overnight. It will take time and refinement, and will need to be reviewed periodically for effectiveness and appropriateness.

The following planning sheet and guidelines will help you begin your personal program. You can make several copies of the planner so that you can easily modify it. As before, you are offered a sample planner first, and then a blank planner that can be photocopied.

Sample Event: Mom fires her helper after two weeks.

Initial Self-Talk	Emotional Reaction	Dysfunctional Thought Patterns	Restructured Thoughts	New Emotional Reaction
How could she do that to me? She'll never accept any help. What am I going to do now? Everything's a mess now.	Anger Anxiety, fear	Personalization Crystal ball gazing Over-generalization	I know she didn't do that purposely to upset me. It may help if I try to understand her reasoning. Just because she fired this one doesn't mean that no one will work. I'm going to try to be understanding. I will collaborate with her to try to prevent this from happening again and to fix whatever parts we can fix.	I wouldn't say I'm happy, but at least I'm calmer, not panicking, and I'm much less angry.

Guidelines

Stress minimizers are activities that serve as methods of relaxation, and that can be built into your lifestyle on a daily basis.

- Make these stress minimizers a part of your daily schedule. Assign a high priority to them and practice them into a habit. It helps to have a partner, especially at first, because working with another person is motivating, and you will be less likely to break a commitment you've made to your partner.

Sample Personal Stress Management Program
Planning Stress Minimizing Activities

Day	Activity	Time and Place	Partner	Potential Obstacles	Alternate Plan	Check if Finished
MON	Treadmill	6:30-7:15 AM Gym	Mary	sore knee	stationary bike	X
	Bubble bath	8:30-9:00 PM Home	None	None. Planned around it to make sure I have time.		X
TUE	Swim	7:30-8:15 PM Pool	None	Bad weather	Gym—stationary bike or treadmill	X
WED	Relaxation tape	6:30-6:50 AM Home	None	None		X
	Reading or craft	8:30-9:15 PM Home	None	None. Turn on answering machine		X
THUR	Treadmill	6:30-7:15 AM Gym	Mary	Sore knee	stationary bike	X
FRI	Relaxation tape	6:30-6:50 AM Home	None	None		X
	Leisure walk	12-12:30 PM Work	Janet	Don't let there be any!		X
SAT	Swim	10-11:00 AM Pool	None	Bad weather	Gym—stationary bike or treadmill	X
SUN	Hike	10 AM-Noon	Tom	Bad weather	Read Sunday paper	X

Notes: _____

_____

_____

Personal Stress Management Program
Planning Stress Minimizing Activities

Day	Activity	Time and Place	Partner	Potential Obstacles	Alternate Plan	Check if Finished
MON						
TUE						
WED						
THUR						
FRI						
SAT						
SUN						

Notes: _____

_____

_____

_____

_____

- Be creative. Think about current activities in your life, activities you did earlier and would like to do again, and activities you have always wanted to try. Ask others what they do to relax. You will probably need to change or refine your program from time to time.

- Prepare for any obstacles that might get in your way. It helps to have an alternate plan. This is especially true for bad weather (if your stress minimizers are outdoor activities), busy times (such as the holiday season), and days on which you don't feel well or are particularly tired or rushed.

- Remember that your program doesn't have to be elaborate. Just a few minutes of relaxation breathing or guided imagery (see below) will be helpful.

- Try to match your activities to your stress style. For example, if you experience stress in mostly physical ways (increased heartbeat, feeling jittery, stomach problems, pacing), try physical relaxers (exercise, massage, sauna, a hot bath). If, on the other hand, your stress is experienced mostly in mental ways (difficulty concentrating, lots of worrying, rumination, being bothered by unimportant thoughts, difficulty making decisions), then try some mental relaxers (meditation, reading, an absorbing hobby). If your style is mixed, you may want to try a physical activity that also demands mental rigor (competitive sports such as racquetball), or any combination of both mental and physical activities.

- Have realistic expectations of yourself. Start with small changes. Set up rewards for having accomplished your small goals.

Relaxation Techniques

Guided Imagery

Guided imagery is an extremely effective relaxation technique. It is based on an appreciation of the power of mind over body. Your brain is so powerful that when you vividly imagine a situation, your body may react physically as if it were actually in that situation. Here is a quick demonstration of this technique:

Close your eyes and vividly imagine that you have cut a particularly juicy, tart lemon in quarters. You pick up one quarter, and tart juices drip onto your hand. You place the lemon in your mouth, bite into it, and your mouth puckers because it's so tart and juicy.

Most people, when doing this exercise, find themselves salivating. Notice that there is no lemon, only the mind's imagination, and yet a physiological reaction follows. So if you imagine yourself in an anxiety-provoking scenario, your body will react by becoming more tense. If, on the other hand, you imagine yourself in a peaceful scene, your body will react by becoming quite relaxed.

Use the scene that follows, or develop one of your own. If you develop your own, remember to use all of your senses. Tape-recording the scene yourself, or having someone whose voice you like record the tape, will make it easier to follow. If the exercise is recorded, have the speaker pause for a few seconds after each sentence. The more you use this tape, the more effective it will be. It is short enough so that you can take it to work with a personal cassette player and use it during your break.

Picture yourself in a forest. It is a bright and friendly forest. You're alone because you wanted to take a long, pleasant walk. The air around you is cool and pleasant. Trees hang over your head and make the forest cool and shadowy, but there are bright spots of sunshine on the ground where the sun has filtered down through the leaves. You are walking barefoot and the leaves and moss feel good and soft on your feet—like a thick rug. The birds are singing soft, pretty songs in the trees, and the sounds make you very happy and comfortable. You have been walking for a long time and your muscles feel very loose and heavy and relaxed from all the exercise. The leaves feel so soft and pleasant beneath your feet that you want to fall down and just close your eyes and rest. You can barely keep your eyes open when you come to a small stream. It is making a soft, bubbling noise that makes you even more relaxed. Next to the stream is the most beautiful place you have ever seen. It is a little patch of tall, soft grass protected all around by tall trees. It is lit and warmed by sunlight. You see it would be the perfect place to rest. You are so relaxed and loose you can barely walk over to the grassy place. But you do walk over and you sink down to your knees, and then fall gently into the soft, warm grass. Your eyes close and you realize you have never laid in as soft a place in your life. Even your bed is not as soft. You have never been so relaxed. Your eyes are closed and you hear the soft, pleasant bubbling of the stream and the singing of the birds. You are completely relaxed, and every single part of your body, from your toes to the top of your head, is completely loose and limp and very, very comfortable.

Tapes using guided imagery or other relaxation techniques can be purchased at local music stores, bookstores, or from mail-order catalogs.

Abdominal Breathing Exercise

Relaxation breathing is also an effective technique for stress reduction. Follow the instructions below to achieve a state of deep relaxation in a short period of time. Just three minutes of abdominal breathing will usually have a pronounced effect in reducing anxiety.

1. Note the level of tension you're feeling. Then place one hand on your abdomen right beneath your rib cage.

2. Inhale slowly and deeply through your nose into the "bottom" of your lungs—in other words, send the air as low down as you can. If you're breathing from your

abdomen, your hand should actually rise. Your chest should move only slightly while your abdomen expands. (In abdominal breathing, the *diaphragm*—the muscle that separates the lung cavity from the abdominal cavity—moves downward. In doing so, it causes the muscles surrounding the abdominal cavity to push outward.)

3. When you've taken in a full breath, pause for a moment and then exhale slowly through your nose or mouth, depending on your preference. Be sure to exhale fully. As you exhale, allow your whole body to just let go (you might visualize your arms and legs going loose and limp, like a rag doll).

4. Do ten slow, full abdominal breaths. Try to keep your breathing *smooth* and *regular*, without gulping in a big breath or letting your breath out all at once. It will help to slow down your breathing if you slowly count to four on the inhale and then slowly count to four on the exhale. Remember to pause briefly at the end of each inhalation. Count from ten down to one, counting backwards one number with each exhalation. The process should go like this:

   Slow inhale . . . Pause . . . Slow exhale (count "ten"), Slow inhale . . . Pause . . . Slow exhale (count "nine"), Slow inhale . . . Pause . . . Slow exhale (count "eight"), and so on down to one. If you start to feel light-headed while practicing abdominal breathing, stop for fifteen to twenty seconds, and then start again.

5. Extend the exercise if you wish by doing two or three sets of abdominal breaths, remembering to count backwards from ten to one for each set.

When to Ask for Professional Help

There are times when it's not just simple stress you're trying to manage. Rather it may be an anxiety disorder. It's important to understand some symptoms of anxiety disorders. Three types of symptoms are indications for seeking professional help. These are

- Panic attacks: episodes of extreme anxiety in which you may experience shortness of breath, rapid heartbeat, nausea, dizziness, feelings of dread, feelings that you might faint, or feelings of derealization.

- Obsessions or compulsions: Obsessions are repetitive thoughts that are anxiety provoking and that you can't get out of your mind. Compulsions are repetitive behaviors you feel driven to repeat that reduce the anxiety for only a short period of time. Common obsessions and compulsions include the need to repetitively check that doors are locked before you leave the house or go to bed, compulsive cleaning, compulsive hand-washing, and obsessive thoughts about sex or violence.

- Any significant symptom of anxiety that lasts more than a couple of weeks without alleviation.

If you have any of these symptoms, you are encouraged to consult a mental health professional. She or he will be able to help you with counseling. In addition, you may require medication to help in the control and resolve these symptoms. Refer to appendix E for help in finding a therapist.

On the following page are ten of the most important tips for stress management. You may want to keep a copy of this at work, on the refrigerator door, or in your day planner.

Summary

- Stress is the reaction that occurs when the demands placed upon us exceed our resources.

- Most people experience a level of stress that is higher than optimal.

- Excess stress can cause negative physical and emotional consequences.

- You can better manage your stress by learning to:

  1. Change the situation.

  2. Change your reaction to the situation.

  3. Increase your tolerance of and preparedness for stress.

Ten Tips for Stress Management

1. Develop realistic expectations and goals for yourself and others.

2. Recognize and acknowledge the small goals you have achieved, instead of criticizing yourself for the goals you haven't achieved.

3. Practice setting appropriate limits on the requests or demands of others. Learn to say "no" respectfully.

4. Make your self-talk constructive.

5. Remember that recreation and leisure are as important and productive as work.

6. Ask for help and learn to delegate. Practice telling your needs and wants to others.

7. Incorporate humor into your life on a regular basis.

8. Listen to yourself and respect your human limitations.

9. Practice a relaxation technique on a daily basis, even if it's only some deep breathing. Do cardiovascular exercise at least three times a week.

10. Separate the things over which you have control from those over which you have no control. Gently and gradually let go of the latter.

13

Communication Skills

With all the changes occurring in your body during midlife, as well as in your partner's, it is important to be able to communicate with your spouse or partner. Talking things out will help you to establish, maintain, and adjust your relationships. If you are not doing so on a regular basis, now is the time to establish good communication with your partner.

This chapter will explore

- Differences in the ways males and females communicate

- Features of good communication, such as empathy and assertiveness

- Tips and exercises for communicating with your partner

This chapter can be helpful, not only for you but also for your partner and family members. Equipped with the skills in these pages, you will all be better prepared to meet the challenges of the midlife years.

Differences in Male and Female Communications

Men and women often misread each other, especially at critical or important times, because of the fundamentally different ways in which they communicate. Your awareness of these differences will increase the success of your efforts to learn about and understand the physical and emotional changes occurring to each of you.

Communication experts have written that men generally engage the world as individual competitors for power and accomplishments. Conversations are aimed at achieving status and keeping the upper hand. Men often feel they need to preserve their independence and need to avoid failure.

Women, on the other hand, tend to approach the world as individuals within a network of relationships. In their world, conversations are negotiations for closeness, and talking is a tool for preserving intimacy. Women often approach problems by talking, not to find solutions, but to seek understanding and empathy. Men, alternatively, tend to approach problems as tasks they are responsible for solving.

There are other male and female differences in communication. For example, when a woman is talking with a man about his feelings, it is important to not misread his quietness as avoidance. Men often need more time than women to get in touch with their feelings. Asking them to respond before they're ready may cause anxiety, which interferes with communication. The eventual result can be a stalemate and withdrawal by both parties. Keeping these differences in mind will help to avoid misunderstandings.

Features of Good Communication

Empathy

When you empathize, you temporarily put aside your own needs and make every effort to understand your partner's point of view. This makes your partner feel heard, validated, and cared for. Your partner is then more likely to work with you in finding a positive solution.

Read the following example for clarification.

John, once again, has become upset that his wife, Betty, is the only one of her four siblings taking care of their aging mother. John feels protective of Betty and feels she is being taken advantage of by her mother's constant demands and her siblings' "convenient" avoidance of their mother. John also feels upset because it takes away from the free time Betty would otherwise have to spend doing things as a couple. Betty, on the other hand, feels it is her responsibility, as the oldest, to provide care for her mother, and she is more comfortable knowing that her mother's needs are being met.

Although John is concerned and feels his needs will be somewhat neglected, he accepts Betty's statement that, "I have told you how I feel about this and I need your support." John is able to temporarily set aside his concerns and personal needs, and to acknowledge the importance to Betty to be there for her mother. He responds, "I realize I get protective of you and upset with your family. I know I am adding more pressure instead of helping to support you, and I apologize. I can understand your feelings, although I have to admit that they're sometimes difficult for me to accept."

Of course, it will also be important for Betty to work on empathizing with John's feelings. In that way, they may be able to find some compromises that work for both of them.

Tips for Empathic Communication

- Listen! An old African proverb states: "He who listens will learn." Be committed to listening even if you are angry and upset.

- Ask "how" and "what" questions: They will help you understand your partner's feelings and thoughts. Try to clarify what you do not understand.

- Leave out "why" questions: They are usually critical and can increase a person's defensiveness (for example, "Why did you slam that door?")

- Don't make assumptions. Verify your impressions so that you can grasp your partner's needs and feelings and not misunderstand them.

- Use "I" messages. That is, begin your statements with the word "I." Starting a sentence with "you" can be perceived as an attack, and the listener is likely to fight back (attack you) or run away (shut down or withdraw).

- Look for areas of agreement. Compromise is the essence of negotiating relationships. No one gets everything he or she wants.

- Try not to be judgmental. Remember, people fear being wrong, and criticism lowers self-esteem.

- Maintain good eye contact.

Assertiveness

When couples communicate, they often use aspects of the three basic styles of communication: passive, aggressive, and assertive. Although assertiveness is usually the goal, there are likely to be instances where you will be aggressive when you feel overwhelmed, or passive when your partner is extremely angry over something you did that was insensitive or hurtful.

Communication with your partner will be at its best when you can identify and understand these three basic styles, because you can then learn to manage them.

Passive means you don't directly express your feelings, thoughts, or wishes. You communicate indirectly with facial expressions or body language, speak softly, or use disclaimers such as, "I'm probably wrong," or "I'm not really sure, but . . ." You discount your opinions or keep them to yourself. You tend to let the other person control the conversation and, at times, control you.

Aggressive means you are very capable of expressing your feelings, wishes, and thoughts, often at the expense of someone else's rights and feelings. You may verbally attack or intimidate the other person to get what you want. You raise your voice and use sarcasm or humorous put-downs. The sentences you use will often begin with "you," rather than "I" and contain absolutes, such as "always" or "never." You are so intent on being right or winning the argument that you don't really hear what others are saying.

Assertive means you make direct statements about your feelings, thoughts, and wishes, while respecting the feelings and rights of others. It also means standing up for your rights and needs. You listen attentively and validate what you are hearing. You are open to negotiations and compromise. Your requests and refusals are direct. Giving and receiving compliments is comfortable. You are capable of hearing criticism and listening for the parts that apply, without responding to it as rejection.

Here is an example of assertive behavior:

Joan needs to speak to her gynecologist, Dr. Mary Dodd, to report concerns about some ongoing physical symptoms she began to notice recently. Dr. Dodd's receptionist does not want to pass on Joan's request until she determines, in her mind, that it is important enough to disrupt Dr. Dodd's extremely busy schedule. Joan, using her assertive abilities, states, "I appreciate your not wanting to interrupt Dr. Dodd right now with all the patients she has scheduled to see today. The doctor and I have talked about these concerns before, and she asked me to call her when they occurred again so she could tell me what steps to take. I will feel much more assured that all is fine once Dr. Dodd and I have spoken personally. I will be home all afternoon today and would appreciate you having the doctor call me back personally, when she is free. Thank you for your help."

An Exercise for Enhancing Your Empathy

The idea behind this exercise is very simple. You are going to act as your partner's defense attorney. Your partner is on trial for behavior that bothers you (something he or she said or did or didn't say or didn't do). You are the attorney and have to persuade the "jury" (really yourself) that what the other person did was, if not right, at least reasonable and understandable from his or her perspective. You are to make as strong a case for your partner as possible. Although it may be hard to believe right now, the stronger the case you make for your partner, the better it will be for you.

You must set your own feelings aside and see the situation as much as possible from your partner's point of view. You can feel free to interview your partner to get information about how he or she feels about and sees the situation.

It is important to take your time and approach this exercise seriously.

When the case material is gathered, you can either present your defense to your partner directly, write it down on paper, or read it into a tape recorder for you to listen to and share if you wish.

Assertiveness Exercise

Below you will find excerpts from three conversations. In the space to the left of each, place an "Ag" if the style is aggressive, a "P" if it is passive, and an "As" if you think it is assertive.

_____ "I'm sorry. I wasn't aware you wanted Italian food tonight. I've already gone shopping and bought fresh fish and vegetables for a salad. I'll make Italian food tomorrow night."

_____ "You never listen to me. You know I was running late tonight and you were supposed to pick the kids up. Now you've gone and ruined my evening again for the third time this week! Don't you ever think?"

"They said it was going to rain today, so maybe we should think about changing our plans to go to the beach. Of course, I could be wrong, so we can still go if you want to."

Now, practice your assertive skills by rewriting the passive and aggressive examples in the spaces below. Sample answers are provided at the end of the exercise.

_____

_____

_____

_____

_____

_____

_____

_____

_____

_____

_____

_____

_____

_____

Possible Answers

"I just heard the weather report stating that there is a good chance of rain. I don't feel like packing all that beach stuff and getting caught in rain. I would prefer waiting for a better day to go to the beach." (Changed from passive.)

"I was under the impression that I told you I would be late tonight. I am upset that the kids were left waiting longer than usual. I would like us to find a way to confirm changes in plans, so we aren't left being upset when we get home." (Changed from aggressive.)

Tips for Asserting Yourself

- Be clear about your goals, needs, or limits before you say anything.

- Treat the other person with kindness and respect.

- When you are angry, stop and cool down so you can talk and listen without defending and attacking.

- Start off with as positive a statement as possible.

- Talk about what you would like or want, rather than what your partner did or did not do that upset you.

- If you must criticize to clarify your point, criticize the behavior, not the person.

- Make the problem yours, as much as possible, rather than your partner's.

- Be as specific as possible about what behavior or information you want.

- Be clear that the request is negotiable, when appropriate. Offer alternative suggestions if you are asking for a change.

- Ask for your partner's understanding of what you said, so you can be sure your words are being correctly interpreted.

Summary

- Communication is one of the most important aspects of any relationship.

- Men and women differ in important ways in their approach to communication. Understanding these differences can enhance communication.

- Learn about and use empathy to increase your ability to listen.

- Be assertive, while decreasing passive and aggressive styles of communication.

14

For Men

This book would be incomplete without a chapter devoted to men, since many men will be learning to cope with menopause along with their female partners. In addition, men are also experiencing changes in midlife that require adjustment. This chapter is written specifically for *men* to read, and will explore

- A crash course in what men need to know about menopause

- Midlife issues for men, including sexual changes and emotional challenges

- The possibility of a male menopause

- Optimizing midlife changes

What Every Man Should Know About Female Menopause

Many men don't know enough to know what to ask about or how to approach the subject of menopause. The more you know about the basics of menopause, the more you will be able to communicate about it with your partner. Here are some frequently asked questions about menopause. For more detailed information you are encouraged to read other sections of this book.

Why does menopause occur?

Women stop menstruating around the age of fifty-one. As a woman ages, the number of her eggs decreases and the remaining ones produce less hormones. With the gradual decrease in estrogen during her early to midforties, a woman often begins to experience many of the signs of menopause. Those signs can include hot flashes, fragmented sleep, night sweats, vaginal dryness, loss of libido, unpredictable or heavy bleeding, stress urinary incontinence, and mood swings. It is important to remember that these are normal experiences for most women.

It is also important to remember that there is no such thing as a "typical menopause" and that all of the changes are genuine and will deserve your support and acceptance.

How long does menopause last?

It is important to remember that, like any other life transition, menopause is temporary. It can last from as few as a couple of years to as many as fifteen years. Like all transitions, it can challenge the patience of both you and your partner at times.

In addition to the physical changes of menopause, your partner may begin to struggle with issues such as the effects of aging, sexual attractiveness, aging parents, employment, and interests outside the family. Most women, however, come through this life transition with increased feelings of self-confidence and a renewed positive outlook on life.

What are hot flashes?

Hot flashes are a physiological reaction that occur when a woman's body temperature increases by as much as seven degrees. In addition, her pulse increases and she begins to perspire, sometimes profusely. The hot flashes generally last only a few minutes. Although most women will experience them, only 10 to 15 percent will find them disruptive enough to cause serious distress. The majority of women will continue to experience them on and off for more than a year, and almost 25 percent will continue to experience them for more than five years.

Hot flashes not only affect women, but they will also affect you. They may keep both of you up at night with the need to change the sheets, adjust the thermostat, or as a result of restless sleep. This often leads to symptoms of sleep deprivation, such as exhaustion, crankiness, memory and concentration difficulties, and irritability for both of you. During this time, you can help your mate by keeping the bedroom cool. Fortunately, hot flashes eventually stop.

How will menopause influence our sex life?

As research suggests, sexual desires with menopausal women can either increase or decrease. The positive changes often come about as a result of the ability to be sexual without contraception. Some women become more relaxed and adventurous. On the other hand, a formerly satisfying and active sex life can be radically changed. Some negative changes may occur when a woman's vagina fails to lubricate as readily, and the skin becomes thinner and easier to tear. This often results in painful intercourse for your partner. The good news is that these changes are often reduced or reversed with regular sexual activity and estrogen hormone replacement therapy. An additional menopausal factor that can interfere in your sex life may be a reduced or complete lack of interest on the part of your partner. It is important to remember that loss of sexual drive or interest is not unusual, and it is not necessarily a reflection on you as a partner, or your sexual attractiveness.

Perhaps the most productive and simplest way to cope with any changes in your sex life is to communicate with your partner about them. There is no reason to assume that menopause means the end of your sex life.

Does menopause make women moody?

Despite common misconceptions and jokes, menopause does not cause depression or "craziness" in women. It also does not mean that your partner's personality will change forever. On the other hand, there are definite chemical changes in a woman's body due to the hormonal fluctuations occurring during menopause. These changes may be associated with mood changes, or an increase in the severity of PMS. It is important to remember that the mood swings your partner may be experiencing are not manipulative. Again, these changes are not permanent.

What issues are of the highest concern to women?

Heart disease. This is the number one cause of death in women after menopause. Postmenopausal women are at a significantly higher risk for cardiovascular disease than their premenopausal counterparts.

Osteoporosis. One out of every three postmenopausal women will develop osteoporosis, increasing their risk for spinal and hip fractures as well as other debilitating conditions.

Hormone replacement therapy. The single biggest controversy associated with menopause is whether or not women should take hormone replacement therapy.

What can I do to help?

As with any major transition or change your partner experiences, the most helpful thing you can do is to be accepting, supportive, and patient. This can be a very difficult time for a woman. Your ability to put your own concerns temporarily on hold, while positively assisting your partner through the ups and downs of menopause, will be helpful. It will also be important to verbalize often that you truly care and still find her attractive.

Midlife Issues for Men

Although there are issues that need to be negotiated during midlife, as in any other stage of the life cycle, there are also positive gains that you can make in self-worth. Midlife is often a time when people reevaluate the choices they have made. While this transition may lead to some turmoil, it can also lead to a sense of feeling more alive and involved with your life.

The following sections of this chapter will first explore sexual changes that may occur for men in midlife, and then focus on the psychological and emotional reactions that may occur, either in reaction to these changes, or as a result of other midlife factors.

Sexual Changes

The two most common changes associated with this time of life are an increase in the time necessary to achieve an erection and occasional failure to achieve an erection. Your penis may not get as full or as firm as before. It is easier for your penis to lose its hardness and, once lost, the hardness may be more difficult to regain. You may experience delayed orgasm or even a failure to achieve an orgasm. The force of your ejaculation will be reduced. Semen may seem to seep out, instead of shoot out. You may also require more stimulation of your penis and other erogenous zones. In most cases, these are just normal changes and nothing to worry about. Many men mistakenly believe that impotence is caused by aging. That is not the case. Impotence or a loss of sexuality is not a consequence of aging, but can be a consequence of one's attitude toward sexuality. Even if you experience some sexual changes, it doesn't mean your level of desire will decrease.

If you are experiencing more serious sexual difficulties, it's important to find the cause. Alcohol is a major contributor to sexual problems. In small amounts it can increase desire. However, in larger amounts or with long-term use, it can cause problems with erection, decreased sexual drive, and ejaculation and orgasmic intensity. Further, medications that you may be taking for depression, anxiety, high blood pressure, or your heart can affect your sexual response.

There are a number of medical conditions known to affect the blood flow to the penis, such as diabetes, heart disease, and hormonal imbalances. It is important to remember that not all erectile problems are in your head. However, some are. Performance anxiety, depression, and relationship problems can certainly interfere with sexuality. If you are having problems, talk to your physician. If the problems are psychological in nature, working with a therapist can be extremely helpful. As always, accurate information is essential, and several books, including an excellent sourcebook entitled *The New Male Sexuality*, by Bernie Zilbergeld, Ph.D., are listed in appendix E.

Is There a Male Menopause?

There are changes occurring in men as they get older that parallel the changes that are occurring in women. However, these physical changes are much milder than those that occur in women. There are hormonal shifts; but, while a woman loses much of her capacity to produce estrogen, a man will only lose his capacity to produce testosterone at a rate of 1 percent per year. Nevertheless, the following are some terms that you may hear in connection with a "male menopause."

While most men will have only minor changes in their testosterone level, researchers estimate that between four and five million men suffer from a significant shortage of testosterone, and that testosterone levels for some men may decline up to 40 percent beginning in their late forties. The symptoms of testosterone deficiency include a loss of sexual desire, fatigue, depression, and osteoporosis. The FDA has recently approved a prescription patch to treat the deficiency: SmithKline Beecham's Androderm is a patch that delivers testosterone over a twenty-four-hour period. Government-sponsored studies are now exploring the use of testosterone supplements that would be used in much the same way as estrogen therapy is used for menopausal women.

Table 14.1
Terms to Know about Male Menopause

Andropause	A term commonly used in Europe and some medical literature. The root of andropause, "*andro*," is Greek for "man."
Viropause	A term gaining use in the media. "*Vir*" is the Latin prefix for "man."
Male Climacteric	Like the female climacteric, this identifies the physical changes at the midlife. It comes from the Greek word, "*klimax*," meaning "ladder."

Psychological and Emotional Issues

While you may or may not experience sexual changes, you will definitely experience other changes that are secondary to aging. You will also have psychological and emotional tasks to master, as you have in other stages of the life cycle.

Your psychological reaction to the normal changes of aging, like the slight decrease in sexuality, can be disturbing enough to interfere with your mental and physical health. At least 15 to 25 percent of all men will experience significant symptoms of sadness, irritability, anxiety, and a sense of personal inadequacy. If you are ambitious, driven, and successful, you are more at risk for developing these problems. In addition, if your expectations of what your life would be like are quite different from reality, you are also at increased risk for developing problems.

Another group of men who have difficulty in midlife are those who place a high value on their appearance. This group may find it very hard to cope with the physical changes midlife brings. The higher the value you put on appearance, the greater the changes of midlife are likely to disturb you. Some men may be thrown into a state of despair by seeing the irreversible changes of aging.

Following is a checklist of reactions that men may experience in midlife. It will be helpful to be aware of these reactions, so that if they do occur, they don't take you by surprise.

Male Midlife Symptom Checklist

1. ____   Feelings of reduced masculinity

2. ____   Increased worry about strength and virility

3. ____   Increased mental fatigue

4. ____   A generalized sense of ill-being or discontent

5. ____   Increased uncertainty about your self-worth or adequacy

6. ____   Confusion about priorities

7. ____   Mood changes not previously experienced, such as irritability or feeling short-tempered

8. ____   Sleep disturbance or insomnia

9. ____   Increase in psychosomatic symptoms, such as headaches or stomach problems

10. ____   Increase in worrying and fearfulness

11. ____   Seeking new, younger friends or youthful wardrobe

12. ____   New sporty cars when this has not been your previous style

13. ____   Increase in poor financial decisions

If you checked more than two or three items, you may want to discuss them with your doctor or a therapist.

Retirement

As you reach middle age, retirement becomes an important issue. For most men, productivity and success in their work is a major contributor to their identity and self-esteem. As a result, the idea of retirement can be a frightening prospect, resulting in a sense of emptiness or worthlessness. In order to make retirement a positive part of your life, your plans for retirement should be actively included in your overall life-planning.

Not only is it important to plan for your retirement, but it is also important to include your partner in your plans. Frequently, especially in more traditional relationships, women will leave financial matters to their husbands, and know very little about them. Since most men are older than their wives and since the average age of widowhood is in the midfifties, it is important that your wife understands your financial affairs and what to do in the event of your death. Having a will is very important, so that if something should happen to you, your estate does not go into probate. It may be important for you and your partner to discuss these issues with an attorney and your financial consultant. While you may not want to think about these matters this far in advance, planning will help you feel that you are taking action and will help you maintain a sense of self-worth. You will be less likely to experience the adverse effects of midlife.

Reassessing Your Goals

Since disappointment that arises because of unrealistic goals is one common cause of negative reactions to midlife, it is important to review and realistically modify the goals set earlier in your life. You may have been taught to expect yourself to reach a certain level of status and economic success by a certain age, like Bill in the following example. If you don't reach it, you feel you are a failure.

Bill Morrison is a department head for a small but successful manufacturing business founded by his father, who is an engineer. Although Bill is very bright and capable, he was always a hands-on type of learner. He never went on to complete his college degree, but jumped right into learning his father's business and making important contributions to production. Over the years, Bill's abilities became well known to many of the company's customers, and he was highly regarded as one of the important assets at the company. Yet, when Bill was in his early fifties, his father retired, and the company was bought out by a larger firm. At that time, Bill was faced with concerns about his future in a large, complex company that did not necessarily appreciate his unique strengths.

In talking with his wife, Lisa, Bill was suddenly faced with wondering if he had really been successful in his life. In comparing himself to his father, a college-educated professional, founder and owner of his own business, and holder of a number of patents, Bill began to feel he hadn't succeeded because he had failed to live up to what his father had accomplished. Lisa listened empathically and was able to help Bill appreciate the accomplishments he had made using his strengths. She was able to point out the importance of the time he spent with her and their children over the years, unlike his father, who was absent in Bill's childhood. She also showed Bill how much in demand he was now from former customers of his father's business. Although Bill knew that Lisa was correct, it took some time for him to be able to reevaluate that message that men have often been taught: "To be a winner, you have to be the one on top and not be satisfied with being successful at your own level."

Tips for Coping with Male Midlife Changes

- Set aside some quiet time in which you take a daily walk, a short trip, or just reflect on what matters to you.

- Look at your goals and decide if they are what you want, or if they only reflect what someone else expects of you. Think about what will make you happy. If you need to modify your current goals, you are not a failure. When you adjust your goals to better fit reality, you are much more likely to be happy.

- Preparing for retirement is essential. Those who plan ahead are less likely to succumb to a lost sense of self-worth.

- Optimize your health by:

  1. Eating a healthy diet

  2. Exercising appropriately

  3. Eliminating smoking

  4. Moderating your alcohol intake

  5. Obtaining adequate medical care for increased blood pressure, heart disease, and any other medical conditions

- Communicate well with your partner. Understanding each other will help you both.

To help you review and revise your goals, try the exercise at the end of the chapter.

Summary

- There are several basic facts about menopause that you, as men, need to know.

- The more you know, and the better you communicate, the more easily you and your partner will be able to cope with this transition as a team.

- There are a number of sexual changes that you may experience that are associated with midlife. The more information you have about these changes, the more easily you will be able to accept them.

- There are also emotional changes that may be associated with midlife, such as questioning your priorities, or experiencing feelings of inadequacy.

- Retirement may present its own challenges, as work has probably been an important part of your identity and self-esteem.

- These midlife challenges can be met, and you can emerge from them with a more solid sense of identity.

Reworking Your Goals

Think back to early adulthood, and try to remember how you envisioned your goals for your life at your current age. Below, a variety of areas are listed in which you may have had goals. After each, write down your previous goal. To the left of each item, rank the order of importance to you at that time (with "1" being most important).

_____ Occupational _____

_____

_____ Financial _____

_____

_____ Physical _____

_____

_____ Emotional _____

_____

_____ Family & close relationships _____

_____

_____ Educational _____

_____

_____ Others (e.g., spiritual, use of leisure time, community participation)

_____

_____

Now review the goals you wrote. Some of them may no longer be feasible or realistic, some may never have been your goals (but rather were goals someone else imposed on you), and some may have changed in their level of importance.

Rewrite some goals for yourself now, which are more realistic. You may not have a goal for every area. Then, rank the order of importance of each of these goal areas. Finally, try to identify one small step you can take in the near future toward attaining each of these goals.

____ Occupational _____

_____

Action Step: _____

_____

____ Financial _____

_____

Action Step: _____

_____

____ Physical _____

_____

Action Step: _____

_____

____ Emotional _____

_____

Action Step: _____

_____

____ Family & Close Relationships _____

_____

(continued on next page)

Action Step: _____

_____

_____ Educational   _____

_____

Action Step: _____

_____

_____ Others (e.g., spiritual, use of leisure time, community participation)

_____

Action Step: _____

_____

If you like, it may be useful to share this with your partner to get her reaction or feedback. It would be a good opportunity to communicate about these issues and obtain support for your endeavors.

15

Putting It All Together

Now that you have become more aware of the issues facing women in menopause, you are better able to see it as a normal biological transition. The next step is to develop a plan or program along with the aid of your health care providers, and adhere to it.

In this chapter, you will

- Collect information to prepare you for discussions with your health care provider(s)

- Develop a plan to take charge of your lifestyle

- Learn an exercise for improving communication with your partner regarding midlife changes

- Develop a personalized approach to optimizing mood, reducing stress, and coping with emotional challenges

- Assemble your menopause resources

Information for Your Visits with Health Care Providers

In this section, checklists, charts, and lists of questions from throughout the book have been included that you can take to your health care team in order to get the best help available. You are encouraged to make several copies of each before you complete it. There are also some tips for communicating with your doctor.

Menstrual Cycle Calendar

Month _____

SUN		MON		TUE		WED		THUR		FRI		SAT	

Directions:

1. Mark each day of your period by placing a diagonal line across the box.

2. For each day of your period, record your level of bleeding.

       "B=L" indicates light bleeding

       "B=M" indicates moderate bleeding

       "B=H" indicates heavy bleeding

3. If there were any days during which you had spotting, record an "S."

4. If you can estimate when ovulation occurred, mark that date with an "O."

5. If there were any days during which you experienced moodiness or mood swings, record an "M."

6. Create other symbols for your own use:

       ___ = _____

       ___ = _____

Hot Flash Chart

Month/Week From: _____ **To:** _____

	SUNDAY	MONDAY	TUESDAY	WEDNESDAY	THURSDAY	FRIDAY	SATURDAY
#1	T: Intensity: Possible Causes:	T: Intensity: Possible Causes:	T: Intensity: Possible Causes:	T: Intensity: Possible Causes:	T: Intensity: Possible Causes:	T: Intensity: Possible Causes:	T: Intensity: Possible Causes:
#2	T: Intensity: Possible Causes:	T: Intensity: Possible Causes:	T: Intensity: Possible Causes:	T: Intensity: Possible Causes:	T: Intensity: Possible Causes:	T: Intensity: Possible Causes:	T: Intensity: Possible Causes:
#3	T: Intensity: Possible Causes:	T: Intensity: Possible Causes:	T: Intensity: Possible Causes:	T: Intensity: Possible Causes:	T: Intensity: Possible Causes:	T: Intensity: Possible Causes:	T: Intensity: Possible Causes:
#4	T: Intensity: Possible Causes:	T: Intensity: Possible Causes:	T: Intensity: Possible Causes:	T: Intensity: Possible Causes:	T: Intensity: Possible Causes:	T: Intensity: Possible Causes:	T: Intensity: Possible Causes:

Directions:

1. Record the time of your hot flash.

2. Rate its intensity from 1–10, with higher numbers indicating greater severity.

3. Note any possible causes—anything you did or experienced that could have precipitated the flash. Choose from the following list, using the highlighted letters in each word as a code:

Alcohol	**C**igarette	**E**xercise	**H**eavy Clothing	**H**ot Food
Forgot **HRT**	**N**ight	**S**tress	**S**picy Food	**W**arm Environment

Others (add your own): _____

4. If you wish to record more than four hot flashes per day, simply photocopy this chart.

The Decision to Take Hormones

How disabling are your menopausal changes? None Mild Moderate Severe
(from table 3.3)

	Yes	No
Do you have:		
Heart disease?	_____	_____
Risk factors for heart disease?	_____	_____
Osteoporosis?	_____	_____
Risk factors for osteoporosis?	_____	_____
Breast cancer?	_____	_____
Are you concerned about endometrial cancer?	_____	_____
Do you have a family history of:		
Cancer?	_____	_____
Heart Disease?	_____	_____
Osteoporosis?	_____	_____
Do you have medical conditions that make HRT inadvisable?	_____	_____
Are you willing to take medication regularly?	_____	_____
Have you considered alternatives to HRT?	_____	_____
Are you willing to:	_____	_____
Eat well?	_____	_____
Exercise regularly?	_____	_____
Stop smoking?	_____	_____
Maintain a desirable weight?	_____	_____
Keep cholesterol under control?	_____	_____
Keep blood pressure under control?	_____	_____
Maintain low caffeine and alcohol intake?	_____	_____

After you have answered these questions for yourself, you will be in a better position to discuss HRT with your physician. Remember, any choice you make is not irrevocable and can be changed in the light of new research information or as alternative treatments become available.

Communicating with Your Doctor

It is essential to feel comfortable talking with your doctor about any questions or concerns you have. If you are intimidated easily, it may be helpful to review some of the information on assertiveness in chapter 13. If you are not satisfied with the care you are receiving, you have the right to change doctors. The importance of having a health care provider who is willing to work with you cannot be over emphasized.

- Make a list of the questions, concerns, and symptoms about which you wish to talk to your doctor.

- Prioritize your list, so that if time is limited, you will be sure to address the most pressing items first.

- Find out before your visit how much time the doctor can spend with you. (This is particularly important in today's changing medical practices, where managed care requirements limit a doctor's time to listen and talk to patients.)

- Find out the level of expertise your doctor has with menopause.

- Take along paper and a pencil so you will be able to record your doctor's answers and review them later.

- Make sure you understand what the doctor is saying to you. If you do not understand a medical term, ask for clarification. For further information, look at the sample list of questions on the following page.

Making the Decision for Hysterectomy

If surgery is recommended for abnormal bleeding, do not feel pressured into doing it. Before agreeing, you should always get a second opinion. Questions you should ask your physician include:

- Can we give it more time to see if the problem clears up on its own?

- What will happen if I choose to do nothing?

- Can the problem be managed with medication?

- Are there any alternatives to surgery?

If you need a hysterectomy, it is important to find a gynecologist who is experienced in doing the procedure. You should ask:

- Is it a vaginal or abdominal hysterectomy?

- How long will the procedure take?

- How long will I be in the hospital?

- What kind of anesthesia will be used?

- What are the possible complications?

- How much will it cost and does that include the follow-up care?

- How long will it take to recover, and what will the recovery period be like?

- When can I start having sex again?

What to Ask Your Doctor About Medication

- What are the possible side effects and risks?

- How long will it be before the medication begins to help?

- Do I have to eat or avoid eating when I take this medicine?

- Will it affect my ability to work, drive, or operate machinery?

- Should I call you if any particular side effects develop?

- Is there any danger from skipping a dose? From taking a double dose?

- Does this medicine interact with any other medications, including over-the-counter medicines?

- Are there any foods or substances, such as alcohol, that I should avoid?

- How long will I have to take this medication?

- What are the alternatives to using this drug?

- What if this drug doesn't work?

Source: *Caring for the Mind*, Diane Hales and Robert E. Hales, M.D. Copyright 1995 by Dianne Hales and Robert E. Hales, M.D. Used by permission of Bantam Books, a division of Bantam Doubleday Dell Publishing Group, Inc.

Lifestyle Changes

Maintaining a healthy lifestyle is what much of this book is about. A healthy heart ensures a longer, more active life. The same can be said of healthy bones. Chapters 4 and 8 identified risk factors and recommended lifestyle changes to help reach the goal of healthier living. Although your first attempts may not be successful, using the flow sheets and charts in this section will help you get back to your goals and help you stay on track. You may want to make several copies for future use.

Also included is a section on sex and communication, since they are the core of a healthy relationship.

Exercise, Nutrition, Caffeine, Alcohol, Smoking

One of the best ways to make changes in your lifestyle is to set small goals that aren't drastic. For example, rather than suddenly decide to go to an aerobics class seven days a week, start with twenty minutes of walking every other day. Changes made gradually are more likely to become permanent.

Below is a list of areas in which you may want to set some specific goals. Make sure the goals are small and specific. You do not need to set a goal under every item. Look at the examples first. Set a date to review the goals. If you aren't consistently reaching them, you may need to revise them. When you begin to achieve these goals consistently, you will again want to review and rewrite them so that they will be more advanced.

Sample: Nutrition

1. To lower my fat intake, I will:

    a) *Use nonfat salad dressing* Review date: *March 15*

    b) *Eat fish instead of red meat twice a week* Review date: *March 15*

2. To increase my calcium intake, I will:

    a) *Eat one serving of nonfat yogurt three times a week* Review date: *March 15*

    b) *Take a calcium/vitamin D supplement five times a week* Review date: *March 15*

Now try it on your own.

Exercise

1. To increase my bone strength, I will:

    a) _____ Review date: _____

    b) _____ Review date: _____

2. To increase my endurance/cardiovascular health, I will:

    a) _____ Review date: _____

    b) _____ Review date: _____

3. To increase my flexibility, I will:

    a) _____ Review date: _____

    b) _____ Review date: _____

Nutrition

1. To lower my fat intake, I will:

   a) _____   Review date: _____

   b) _____   Review date: _____

2. To increase my calcium intake, I will:

   a) _____   Review date: _____

   b) _____   Review date: _____

You may want to add other nutrition goals. Use the space at the bottom of the page.

Caffeine

1. To reduce my caffeine intake, I will:

   a) _____   Review date: _____

   b) _____   Review date: _____

Alcohol

1. To reduce my alcohol intake, I will:

   a) _____   Review date: _____

   b) _____   Review date: _____

Smoking

1. To reduce my cigarette intake, I will:

   a) _____   Review date: _____

   b) _____   Review date: _____

Other goals

   _____   Review date: _____

   _____   Review date: _____

   _____   Review date: _____

   _____   Review date: _____

   _____   Review date: _____

Sex and Communication

On pages 157 and 158, you will find charts concerning psychological and physical changes that may occur during menopause and midlife. Please go over the lists and place a check next to any changes you are experiencing. Ask your partner to do the same. Next, go back and rank the changes (on a scale of 1 to 10) you are most concerned about, or would most like to discuss with your mate (with "1" being the most important). Then, exchange lists with your mate and review the changes and concerns your mate identified. Finally, as a couple, review the chapters that discuss the particular areas each of you have checked as concerns. If you find you need or would like additional information or help, please see the Resources section in appendix E for more references.

Psychological Changes—Male and Female

Rank	Changes	Yes
_____	Concerns about physical attractiveness (thinning hair, muscle tone, etc.)	_____
_____	An increase in sexual interest	_____
_____	A decrease in sexual interest	_____
_____	Increased pressure to provide for mate and/or family	_____
_____	Increased avoidance of mate and family	_____
_____	Decreased or plateauing professional/career growth	_____
_____	Increased symptoms of stress or anxiety	_____
_____	Increased symptoms of depression	_____
_____	Increased intake of alcohol or drugs (prescription or not)	_____
_____	Fatigue	_____
_____	Boredom	_____
_____	Concerns about health changes or illness	_____
_____	Concerns about mortality	_____
_____	Concerns about financial security	_____
_____	Other:	_____
_____	Other:	_____

Physical Changes—Female

Rank	Changes	Yes
_____	Takes longer to get arouse	_____
_____	Arousal is less intense	_____
_____	Orgasm is shorter or less intense	_____
_____	Vaginal dryness	_____
_____	Painful uterine contractions during or after intercourse	_____
_____	Irregular or no periods	_____
_____	Premenstrual symptoms	_____
_____	Hot flashes	_____
_____	Insomnia	_____
_____	Headaches	_____
_____	Problems with memory	_____
_____	Other:	_____

Physical Changes—Male

Rank	Changes	Yes
_____	Takes longer to attain an erection	_____
_____	Takes longer to reach an ejaculation	_____
_____	Ejaculations are less forceful	_____
_____	Time between ejaculations is longer	_____
_____	Erections lose their firmness quickly after ejaculation	_____
_____	Require longer and more varied stimulation to regain a lost erection	_____
_____	Problems with memory	_____
_____	Other:	_____

Emotional Issues and Stress Management

As in any phase of life there can be significant psychological changes with which we have to deal. The emotional issues create challenges that in the best sense can allow us to grow. Meeting these challenges, in part, depends on good, supportive interpersonal relationships, along with other resources. Following the tips and suggestions in this book can help you negotiate the tides of change with the reward of increased self-understanding, acceptance, and confidence.

You have already learned how to use the exercises reprinted at the end of this chapter for maximizing mood and reducing stress. You might want to look back at chapters 11 and 12 to review their use. Again, make photocopies prior to completion for future use of these exercises.

Assembling Your Menopause Resources

The next section of this chapter addresses how to assemble your menopause team. It will include how to choose a doctor, how to find a therapist if you are experiencing psychological difficulties, the use of support groups, and taking advantage of other resources.

How to Find Health Care Professionals

The American Psychological Association prints a pamphlet on how to find a competent psychotherapist, and the local psychiatric society can recommend a psychiatrist. Here are some ideas to keep in mind:

- Ask your physician or friends for trusted referrals.

- Make sure the professional is licensed by the state.

- Talk to the psychotherapist/psychiatrist before scheduling an appointment.

- Feel free to ask the psychotherapist/psychiatrist if your area of concern is an area of specialty for him or her. Ask about his or her approach. Some mental health professionals will be willing to talk with you in person for a brief time without charge.

Your choices in the selection of a physician may be limited by your insurance plan. However, following are some tips that may be helpful in your selection process:

- Ask friends who have the same insurance plan for the names of doctors they recommend.

- Ask other medical professionals such as a pharmacist, nurse at a hospital, or your primary care physician for recommendations.

- Call a local medical society or nearby university medical center for a referral.

- Ask your church or synagogue for names.

- When asking for a recommendation, specify whether you prefer a male or female.

Support Groups

Belonging to a support group can be beneficial for a number of reasons. Whether the support group deals specifically with the transitions involved in menopause, general women's issues, or some particular subject that is more relevant to you (such as depression, anxiety, or smoking cessation) you can hope to obtain the following benefits from participation:

- Education about a variety of pertinent topics

- Support and understanding from others about your experiences

- Information about available resources

- Reduced feelings of isolation

- Good ideas for solving common problems

- Hope and optimism

- A potential source of new friends with whom you may share much in common

- An additional activity, to help optimize your mood

There may already be existing support groups for menopause or related topics in your area. You can learn about them from your local newspaper, a local or national information and referral line, your health care providers, or others who are having experiences similar to you. It is important to remember that not every group is constructive or helpful. If there is more than one group for a particular topic in your area, you will probably want to try each of them to see which best fits your preferences with regard to style or participants.

Some support groups are leaderless, some have a lay facilitator, and some are led by a professional. No matter who leads the group, avoid groups where:

- People are overly critical of others

- The focus is only on the negative

- Certain individuals dominate the discussion for long periods of time, preventing others from participating

If there is not a support group in your area, you might consider starting one. Begin by arranging a time and place (often churches and hospitals will allow you free use of a room if you are not charging for participation), asking people who you think might be interested in participating, and advertising in the local newspaper(s) and radio station(s). These advertisements are frequently free of charge. Make sure to tell your health care providers so that they can pass on the information to other patients. At the first group meeting, you can, as a group, make some decisions regarding time and frequency of meetings, guidelines for group process and format, and address financial issues if money is required for a speaker, flyers, or educational materials. Good luck!

Using Resources

At this point you may want to refer to appendix E for the different resources available to you. These include book titles and the names of organizations that offer information, referrals, pamphlets, and hot lines. Be aware that each group may have different slants and approaches to menopause. You need to decide which ones are most compatible with your perspective.

Midlife Challenges

Below is a list of commonly experienced changes that may occur during midlife. Check all that apply to you.

_____ Entry, re-entry, or exit from the workforce

_____ Change in job, career, or income

_____ Being a member of the "sandwich generation"—caring for family members in the older and younger generations simultaneously

_____ "Empty Nest"/"Return to the Nest"—coping with adult children who have left or returned home

_____ Becoming a grandparent

_____ Loss of a significant other or family member, through death, divorce, or other circumstances

_____ Becoming single or entering new relationships

_____ Change in appearance

_____ Concerns about illness and mortality

_____ Reevaluation of priorities

Now pick two or three of these changes and set personal goals for coping with them. Photocopy the list before setting your initial goals so that you will be able to use it as necessary.

Goal: _____

_____

Action Step: _____

_____

Goal: _____

_____

Action Step: _____

_____

Goal: _____

_____

Action Step: _____

_____

Each month, evaluate your success in meeting these goals and formulate new or revised goals if appropriate.

Five Column Technique				
Initial Self-Talk	Emotional Reaction	Dysfunctional Thought Patterns	Restructured Thoughts	New Emotional Reaction

Activity Schedule
Day:_____

Time	Activity	Companion	Reward	Check if Done

Personal Stress Management Program
Planning Stress Minimizing Activities

Day	Activity	Time and Place	Partner	Potential Obstacles	Alternate Plan	Check if Finished
MON						
TUE						
WED						
THUR						
FRI						
SAT						
SUN						

Notes: _____

_____

_____

_____

_____

Epilogue

Now that you've learned more than any previous generation has about menopause, what greater gift can you share with your own daughters than your newfound knowledge? Below is a sample letter we have written, sharing our thoughts and feelings about menopause. You may want to write your own.

Letter to My Daughter

I am glad I can speak openly to you about menopause and to pass on to you the lessons that I have learned. While for many who have gone before me, this transition was marked with mystery and fear, I hope that your experience will be different and that you can speak openly about what is happening to you and your body and accept it as part of everyday life.

I hope to prepare you for this by helping you learn to care for yourself. This includes taking care of your body by eating a healthy diet with plenty of calcium, enjoying your body with regular exercise, and being accepting of yourself and your feelings. I hope that my openness with you will also be a part of your relationship with your partner and family, so that you can support each other through the changes that will happen to both of you during this time.

I hope that you will respect yourself so that you will experience this change, not as a loss of your femininity, but as a ripening into a mature woman who has mastered much of what life has to offer, and who will continue to see challenges and growth for herself in the future.

Lastly, I hope you appreciate your opportunity to take more direct control of your life and your body, and to have an active say in your medical support. Please remember you will be able to do this with the knowledge that you can always ask me or your father for our support when and if you need it.

A

Important Medical Tests for Women Before and During Menopause

Tests That Should Be Done Regularly

Monthly

Breast self-exam. Women should do this once a month for life. Ten percent of cancers that are not picked up by mammogram are picked up by breast self-examination. A description of how this is done is included in appendix B.

Annually

Bimanual (pelvic) exam for ovarian cancer, ovarian cysts, and uterine tumors. The exam should be done to insure that the uterus is of normal size and that the ovaries have no cysts or tumors. This exam needs to be done annually even after hysterectomy.

Mammograms for breast cancer. This should be performed at age thirty-five and repeated every one to two years until age fifty. After age fifty, yearly screenings should be done. The breast is flattened and an X ray is taken. The procedure lasts four to five seconds per breast and is mildly uncomfortable.

Pap smears for malignant and premalignant conditions of the vagina, cervix, and endometrium. A swab is taken from the vaginal walls and uterine lining. The exam is usually done annually, but may be done for unexplained vaginal bleeding and more frequently if there is a history of herpes, human papilloma virus, or DES exposure. This exam should be continued even after hysterectomy.

Cholesterol/lipid profile. This test will help determine your risk for heart disease.

Every Three to Five Years

Sigmoidoscopy is performed to detect colon cancer. Women over fifty should have this done. It will allow your physician to see whether you have polyps in the lower portion of the colon. Since polyps can exist for five to seven years before they become malignant, precancerous conditions can be detected. Some physicians will test the stool for occult blood.

Other Diagnostic Tests That May Be Indicated

Follicle stimulating hormone (FSH) is used to measure the estrogen level. The test is done if you are experiencing hot flashes or a changing menstrual pattern. Your physician will be able to tell you whether you are perimenopausal or menopausal by the results of this test.

Estradiol measures blood levels of estradiol. Levels of less than fifty picograms per milliliter are associated with hot flashes, sleep changes, and sexual difficulties.

Ultrasound is performed if there is any question of a pelvic mass. Routine ultrasound is not usually indicated.

Electrocardiograms and stress tests are performed on women who are at risk for heart disease. This includes those with a high cholesterol level, a family history of heart attack before the age of sixty, women who smoke, and women who are hypertensive.

Bone density test measures the bone mineral content. It is performed on women in their forties or fifties who are at risk for osteoporosis. This includes thin white women, smokers, or those who take thyroid medication or steroids, have a history of irregular periods, or have a strong family history of osteoporosis. This test is usually repeated after menopause, especially in women who are not on estrogen, to insure that they are not losing calcium rapidly.

Endometrial or intrauterine biopsy is done to detect endometrial cancer or hyperplasia. This test is done if there is heavy or irregular vaginal bleeding. Tissue from the endometrial lining is collected by suction.

Vaginal smear measures estrogen levels. A swab is taken from the inner third of the side vaginal wall during a routine pelvic exam. If a low estrogen profile is discovered, an FSH will be done to confirm the diagnosis. This test is not as reliable as an FSH level.

Transvaginal sonography measures the thickness of the uterine lining, existing cysts, endometrial hyperplasia, and ovarian cancer. If the thickness of the endometrium is five millimeters or greater, an endometrial biopsy may be required.

Hysteroscopy is a test in which a fiber-optic instrument is inserted into the uterus and a biopsy of uterine tissue can be obtained. The difference between this and an intrauterine biopsy is that, in this procedure, the physician can see the area being biopsied.

B

Breast Self-Examination

The following information has been reprinted with permission from the American Cancer Society. For more information call them toll free at 1-800-ACS-2345. The American Cancer Society's materials and programs are provided free of charge and are supported by public contributions.

Because you are a woman

You need to know certain facts about breast cancer.

First, *all women are at risk* for breast cancer. Breast cancer now causes more deaths among women than any other cancer except lung cancer.

You also need to know that many breast cancers may be curable. But *only* if they are found early.

Keep in mind

That these factors put you at a higher risk for having breast cancer:

- Over age 50

- History of breast cancer in your close family

- First childbirth after age 30

- Never having children

- Obesity (weighing 40% more than your ideal body weight)

Your best defense

Is to find breast cancer early. And when breast cancer is found in its earliest stages, the chance for a cure is greatest.

Decide on a personal plan

So that you can enjoy your good health without worry. With your doctor, set up a plan of action that will include:

- Doctor's exam

- Mammography

- Self-exam

You'll need

To see your health care professional for a *clinical breast exam*. All women over age 20 should have a clinical breast exam once every three years. After the age of 40, have your doctor check your breasts every year.

The most important part of your action plan

Is having regular *mammograms*. These simple breast X rays are quick, easy, and safe. In fact, mammograms use less radiation than a dentist's X ray.

And a mammogram can give you a big head start on treatment. You and your doctor may feel a lump as small as a pea. But a mammogram can detect a cancer as small as a pin head. That may be up to two years before you can feel it.

The American Cancer Society advises you to have your first mammogram by the age of 40. Your doctor will be able to compare this x-ray with future exams. At the age of 40, schedule a mammogram every one to two years.

As you grow older, your chances of having breast cancer will increase. Almost half of all breast cancer occurs in women 65 and older. So, when you reach the age of 50, start having a mammogram each year.

For guidelines on getting an accurate, high-quality mammogram, call this toll-free number: 1-800-ACS-2345.

The third part of your plan

Will be regular, thorough *breast self-examination*. Starting at the age of 20, all women should check their breast for lumps, thickness, or other changes every month.

First, you should check each breast all over and include the armpit. Use your finger pads and go in an up and down motion. Your doctor can teach you the right way to check yourself. You should also look at your breasts in a mirror. Look for any changes in size or shape.

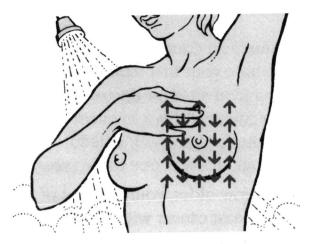

Plan to examine your breasts at the same time every month. It won't take long. And you'll know you've done your part to protect yourself until your next doctor's exam and mammogram.

If you think you have found a lump, see your doctor. Most breast lumps are not cancer, but you won't know if you don't ask.

Your chances are excellent

If you begin your action plan now. We don't yet know how to prevent breast cancer. But we do know how to find it early, when the chance for a cure is greatest.

Put your plan into action right away. Then you can spend your life enjoying your health.

If you are less than 40 years old, the American Cancer Society recommends that you:

- Examine your breasts monthly
- Have a breast exam by your doctor at least every three years

If you are between 40 and 49 years old:

- Examine your breasts monthly
- Have a breast exam by your doctor every year
- Have a mammogram every one to two years

If you are age 50 and over:

- Examine your breasts monthly
- Have a breast exam by your doctor every year
- Have a mammogram every year

C

Discussion of HRT Studies

In attempting to answer the question of whether HRT is effective, you have heard about several different studies. You may want to follow them, particularly the Women's Health Initiative. In this massive study, new data will be generated that will answer many questions about the effectiveness and risks of HRT. If you are interested in participating in this study, please see appendix E, Menopause Resources.

The first study that is often quoted is the Nurses' Health Study (NHS). The NHS includes information from the health records of over 120,000 women over a twenty-year period. It has looked at a wide range of suspected health-related risk factors—from hair dye and hormone replacement therapy to high-fat diets. The NHS tracks the group's health through interviews and questionnaires. Periodically, the gathered data are reviewed with certain questions in mind. For example, in looking at the question of the link between estrogen usage and cancer, the researchers divided the women into two groups: women who reported they had taken estrogen and women who reported they had not. The researchers then compared the two groups. If estrogen has no effect on breast cancer risk, the breast cancer rate in both groups would be the same. If estrogen raises the risk of developing breast cancer, the group taking hormones would have a higher cancer rate. If hormones reduced the risk, this group would have a lower cancer rate.

As you read this book and make decisions about how you will approach menopause and what interventions you will use, it is important to understand a little bit about scientific research. There are many ways to test the safety and efficacy of health treatments.

Without question, and by far the most effective method is that of the *double-blind study* using random selection and placebo. This means that research subjects are randomly selected to take part in the study from the population to whom you want to generalize your results.

Those subjects are then randomly assigned to either the experimental group or the control group. The experimenters are "blind," in that they do not know who is in the control group and who is in the experimental group. The control group receives a *placebo*—treatment that is not expected to have any effect. The experimental group is given the treatment that is being tested. The placebo (which would have inert ingredients) would look just like the real medication, so that no one would be able to know which is which. This is the only way in which we can be sure that the hopes or expectations of the experimenter won't influence the results.

After the treatment is given, the effects are recorded, and the results from the control group are statistically compared to those from the experimental group, to see if the treatment was effective. The larger the number of people studied, the more reliable the results. Having large numbers of people reduces the probability that the differences seen are due to chance alone.

The PEPI Study (Postmenopausal Estrogen/Progestin Intervention study) is one of the few studies that fits the requirement for a double-blind placebo controlled study. It was designed to look at the differences between women who were either using or not using estrogen and progestin. Its purpose was to answer the question of whether HRT benefits might be overstated because women who choose to use HRT are generally healthier and would be expected to have lower rates of heart disease and osteoporosis anyway. The PEPI Study involved 875 healthy postmenopausal women, ages forty-five to sixty-four. Of those women, 278 had undergone hysterectomies. The women were then randomly assigned to one of five treatments: daily estrogen plus natural progesterone for twelve days a month; daily estrogen plus a synthetic progesterone twelve days a month; daily estrogen plus daily progestin; daily unopposed estrogen; or placebo. It was found that at the end of three years, one-third of the women who were on unopposed estrogen had developed endometrial hyperplasia. None of the women who took any estrogen/progestin combination developed this condition. Women who were on natural progesterone had the highest HDL levels. What the study does not answer is the question of whether HRT actually reduces heart disease, because it did not last long enough. The data on osteoporosis will be published later this year.

Whether or not HRT reduces heart attacks, prevents osteoporosis, or increases the risk of breast cancer is currently being studied in the Women's Health Initiative. This study is being conducted by the National Institutes of Health, in a total of forty clinical centers nationwide. It will address the questions of whether HRT diminishes the risk of heart disease and osteoporosis and whether HRT increases breast cancer risk, by carefully following 160,000 women between the ages of fifty and seventy-nine for several years. Each woman will be randomly assigned either to a group receiving a specified intervention or to an untreated control group. The remainder will be enrolled in the observational study, which is designed to yield a large database.

The results of these studies will be much more powerful than those gained from the Nurses' Health Study or from anecdotal evidence. *Anecdotal evidence* is the term used to describe observations by clinicians and their patients on the effectiveness of a treatment, but the data is gathered when everyone knows which treatment is being used and what the expected or hoped for results will be. Furthermore, this type of data can be flawed because it doesn't show what would have happened had the patient not had the treatment. While that does not mean that this type of evidence is meaningless, it suggests that there are opportunities for inaccuracy.

D

The Concept of Risk:
Explaining HRT Statistics

After reviewing the pros and cons of taking hormones, you may be confused about the concept of risk. The term *risk factor* is used to describe a specific practice or physical characteristic that increases the likelihood of disease. For example, smoking is a risk factor for heart disease. Increasing numbers of studies have been done to identify risk factors so that lifestyles can be modified to reduce the chance of developing certain diseases. For instance, if the figures from the Nurses' Health Study are applied to the average fifty-seven-year-old who has been on hormone therapy for more than five years, her risk of developing cancer is 40 percent higher than a similar woman who has not taken hormones, or 0.4 percent. This means that she has a 1 in 292 chance of developing cancer. To put it in perspective for other illnesses, for every one thousand postmenopausal women:

- 10 will develop heart disease

- 3 will develop breast cancer

- 5.5 will develop severe bone loss

- 1.5 will develop endometrial cancer

A large increase in risk of a disease you are unlikely to get may not be nearly as important as a small increase in risk of a disease that you are already at an elevated risk to develop. For example, if you have a positive family history of heart disease, and you already have high blood lipid levels and hypertension, but there is no history of breast cancer in your family, you may not be very concerned about the risk of developing breast cancer on HRT. On the other hand, if you have close family members who have had breast cancer, and you have no family history or risk factors for heart disease, you are likely to be very concerned about the increased risk for breast cancer with HRT, however small the increase.

You do not need to be a statistician when it comes to computing risk. The risk figures will give you the odds of developing a certain problem. Because they are based on populations, they will not tell you what the probability is that *you* will develop or escape a certain illness. However, they can provide general guidelines. Anything that has been identified as a risk factor by several independent investigations is worth taking seriously. A slight elevation (10 to 30 percent) in the risk of a given disease represents only a minor increase in risk. However, a marked increase should be taken seriously. An example of a marked increase would be an increase of 100 percent (which means the risk is doubled) or more.

In the end, our genetic makeup is the strongest single determinant of risk. For most of us, the best indicator of this risk is our personal family history. Therefore, it is important to gather information about the illnesses in your family. Armed with that information, you will be in a better position to make an informed decision about HRT.

E

Menopause Resources

Resources on Alternative Approaches to Health

American Association of Naturopathic Physicians
2366 Eastlake Avenue East
P.O. Box 20386
Seattle, WA 98102
206-323-7610
This organization offers information about the naturopathic approach to health.

American Chiropractic Association
1701 Clarendon Boulevard
Arlington, VA 22209
800-986-4636
This organization offers information about the chiropractic approach to health. They offer a variety of literature on chiropractic health care.

American Holistic Medical Association
4101 Lake Boone Trail, Suite 201
Raleigh, NC 27607
919-787-5146
This organization offers general information about holistic medicine and will provide you with a directory of physicians and osteopaths in your area who use this approach.

American Osteopathic Association
142 East Ontario Street
Chicago, IL 60611
800-621-1773
This organization offers information on the osteopathic approach to health. They will refer you to state organizations who can provide you with names of licensed doctors of osteopathy in your area.

Herb Research Foundation
1007 Pearl Street, Suite 200
Boulder, CO 80302
303-449-2265
This is an organization which sponsors research and education on the use of herbs. They offer information packets on a number of herbal supplements.

National Center for Homeopathy
801 N. Fairfax Street, Suite 306
Alexandria, VA 22314
703-548-7790
This organization will provide you with general information on homeopathy and a directory of practitioners and pharmacies.

National Commission for the Certification of Acupuncturists
P.O. Box 97075
Washington, D.C. 20090-7075
202-232-1404
This organization certifies acupuncturists and Chinese herbologists throughout the United States.

Resources on General Health

Cancer Prevention Information

American Cancer Society
National Office
1599 Clifton Road, NE
Atlanta, GA 30329
800-227-2345
This 800 number will automatically connect you with the regional office. The ACS offers free literature on the early detection of various types of cancer and on smoking cessation, as well as referrals to peer support groups, and to centers which offer low-cost mammography.

National Cancer Institute, Cancer Information Service
Building 31, Room 10A16
Bethesda, MD 20892
800-422-6237
This 800 number is answered regionally by trained cancer information specialists. In addition, they offer publications on a variety of subjects, and referrals to community services and support groups.

Heart and Lung Health

American Heart Association, National Center
7272 Greenville Avenue
Dallas, TX 75231
800-242-8721
This organization offers pamphlets, videotapes, and brochures on heart disease and its prevention. They also offer referrals to support groups in your area.

National Heart, Lung, and Blood Institute, Information Center
P.O. Box 30105
Bethesda, MD 20824-0105
301-251-1222
The NHLBI offers information on the reduction of risk factors and prevention of heart disease. Their fact sheets cover high blood pressure, cholesterol, obesity, heart disease, and cigarette smoking. They also offer a handbook titled *The Healthy Heart Handbook for Women*.

American Lung Association, National Office
1740 Broadway
New York, NY 10019
800-586-4872
When calling this number, you will automatically be routed to your regional office. This organization offers extensive literature on smoking cessation and lung disease, as well as referrals to support groups.

Nutrition

American Dietetic Association
216 West Jackson Boulevard
Chicago, IL 60606-6995
Consumer Nutrition Hotline
800-366-1655
This organization offers recorded food and nutrition messages, answers to food and nutrition questions from a registered dietitian, and referrals to registered dietitians in your area.

Osteoporosis Prevention and Information

National Osteoporosis Foundation
1150 17th Street, NW, Suite 500
Washington, DC 20036-4603
202-223-2226

This organization is dedicated to reducing the incidence of osteoporosis through research, education, and advocacy. They offer a sixty-page handbook with prevention and treatment tips, a quarterly newsletter, access to a patient information center, and the best book for the lay public on osteoporosis: *Boning Up on Osteoporosis: A Guide to Prevention and Treatment.*

Women's Health Initiative

The U.S. Department of Health and Human Services,
Public Health Service, National Institutes of Health
Women's Health Initiative
Federal Building, Room 6A09
Bethesda, MD 20892
800-549-6636

You can become part of this major research study of women and their health if you are between fifty and seventy-nine years of age, past menopause, and planning to live in the same area for at least three years.

Resources on Menopause and Women's Health

A Friend Indeed Publications, Inc.
Box 1710
Champlain, New York 12919-1710
514-843-5730

This newsletter is devoted to support, information, and knowledgeable decision making about menopause. Back issues on a variety of topics are offered.

American Menopause Foundation, Inc.
Madison Square Station
P.O. Box 2013
New York, NY 10010
212-475-3107

This organization is devoted to advocacy, research, and education on menopause. They offer literature, educational programs, support groups, and a newsletter.

Boston Women's Health Book Collective
240-A Elm Street, 3rd Floor
Somerville, MA 02144
617-625-0271
This organization is devoted to women's health education, advocacy, and consulting. They sponsor the Women's Health Information Service and collaborated in the writing of *The New Ourselves, Growing Older: Women Aging with Knowledge and Power.*

Melpomene Institute
1010 University Avenue
St. Paul, MN 55104
612-642-1951
This organization is devoted to the study of women's health and physical activity. They offer a variety of services including a collection of information packets.

Menopause News
2074 Union Street, Suite 10
San Francisco, CA 94123
800-241-6366
This is a subscription newsletter written solely about menopause. It contains medical information both traditional and alternative as well as book reviews and essays. Back issues on a variety of topics are offered.

National Institute on Aging
P.O. Box 8057
Gaithersburg, MD 20898
800-222-2225
The NIA publishes a booklet "Menopause," as well as a fact sheet, "Managing Menopause."

National Women's Health Network
514 10th Street, NW, Suite 400
Washington, DC 20004
202-347-1140
This organization advocates for women in the United States health care system. They offer an extensive clearinghouse of women's health information with packets on over fifty topics, including HRT, alternative therapies, osteoporosis, and heart disease.

National Women's Health Resource Center
2425 L Street, NW, 3rd Floor
Washington, DC 20037
202-293-6045
This is a clearinghouse for women's health information. They offer a bimonthly health report on a variety of women's health issues, reports on such subjects as osteoporosis and HRT, and referrals to women's centers.

North American Menopause Society
P.O. Box 94527
Cleveland, OH 44101
216-844-8748
900-370-6267
This is a nonprofit organization that promotes the understanding of menopause among health care professionals and consumers. They publish a number of booklets as well as a newsletter and a suggested reading list.

Older Women's League (OWL)
666 Eleventh Street, NW, Suite 700
Washington, DC 20001
800-825-3695
OWL promotes equality for midlife and older women in areas including economics, politics, and health. They offer a bimonthly newsletter, as well as publications on topics including heart disease, menopause, and osteoporosis.

Santa Fe Health Education Project
P.O. Box 577
Santa Fe, NM 87504
505-982-9520
This organization publishes the book, *Menopause: A Self-Care Manual,* and offers a bilingual newsletter on health care for women.

Resources on Mental Health and Addictions

Addiction

Alcoholics Anonymous
Your local phone book should have this listing under its Community Services section. Similar twelve-step organizations exist for other addictions.

National Council on Alcoholism and Drug Dependence
800-622-2255
This organization offers information on the treatment of alcoholism and drug dependence.

Nicotine Anonymous
World Service Office
415-750-0328
This organization will refer you to local support groups for smoking cessation.

Rational Recovery Systems
Box 800
Lotus, CA 95651
916-621-4374

Depression

National Foundation for Depressive Illness
P.O. Box 2257
New York, NY 10116
800-248-4344
This organization offers a bibliography and referrals to support groups and physicians in your area.

Referrals for Mental Health Professionals

American Association for Marriage and Family Therapists
1133 15th Street, NW, Suite 300
Washington, DC 20005
202-452-0109

American Psychiatric Association
1400 K Street, NW
Washington, D.C. 20005
202-682-6000

American Psychological Association
750 First Street, NE
Washington, DC 20002-4242
800-374-2721, Referral line: ext. 5800
In addition to referrals, the APA offers a publication entitled "Finding Help: How to Choose a Psychologist."

National Association of Social Workers
1016 23rd Street
Sacramento, CA 95816
800-538-2565

Support Groups

Supportive Older Women's Network (SOWN)
2805 North 47th Street
Philadelphia, PA 19131
215-477-6000
This group assists women over the age of sixty in the formation of support groups. They publish a newsletter that offers guidelines for such groups.

Books and Articles

Alberti, R., and Emmons, M. 1994. *Your Perfect Right*. San Luis Obispo, CA: Impact Publishers.

Bailey, C. 1991. *The New Fit or Fat*. Boston: Houghton Mifflin Company.

Barbarch, L. 1984. *For Each Other: Sharing Sexual Intimacy*. New York: Signet Penguin Books.

Bergman, S.J. 1996. "Male Relational Dread." *Journal of Psychiatric Annals*, Vol. 26, Num. 1.

Bourne, E.J. 1995. *The Anxiety & Phobia Workbook*. Oakland, CA: New Harbinger Publications, Inc.

Brody, J. 1988. *Jane Brody's Nutrition Book*. New York: Bantam Books.

Burns, D.D. 1990. *The Feeling Good Handbook*. New York: Penguin Group.

Burns, D.D. 1985. *Intimate Connections* New York: Penguin Group.

Carrera, M. 1981. *Sex, the Facts, the Acts & Your Feelings*, New York: Crown Publishers.

Colgrove, M., Bloomfield, H., and McWilliams, P. 1991. *How to Survive the Loss of a Love*. Los Angeles: Prelude Press.

Consumer Reports. 1995. "Herbal Roulette." Vol. 60, No. 11, pp. 698–705.

Davis, M., Eshelman, E., and McKay, M. 1995. *The Relaxation & Stress Reduction Workbook*. Oakland, CA: New Harbinger Publications, Inc.

Dowling, C. 1993. *You Mean I Don't Have to Feel This Way?* New York: Bantam Books.

Ellis, A. and Velten, E. 1992. *When AA Doesn't Work for You*. New Jersey: Barricade Books, Inc.

Eshleman, R. 1994. *American Heart Association Cookbook*. New York: Ballantine Books.

Friday, N. 1991. *Women on Top*. New York: Pocket Books, a Division of Simon & Schuster.

Gawain, S. 1982. *Creative Visualization*. New York: Bantam.

Gold, M.S. 1995. *The Good News About Depression: Breakthrough Medical Treatments That Can Work for You*. New York: Bantam.

Gray, J. 1995. *Mars and Venus, in the Bedroom*. New York: HarperCollins Publishers.

Gray, J. 1996. *Mars and Venus, Together Forever*. New York: HarperCollins Publishers.

Gray, J. 1992. *Men Are from Mars, Women Are from Venus*. New York: HarperCollins Publishers.

Hill, A.M. 1993. *Viropause/Andropause, The Male Menopause*. Far Hills, NJ: New Horizon Press.

Ito, D. 1994. *Without Estrogen*. New York: Crown Publishers, Inc.

James, J., and Cherry, F. 1988. *The Grief Recovery Handbook*. New York: Harper & Row.

Krumholz, H.M., and Phillips, R.H. 1993. *No Ifs, Ands or Butts* New York: Avery Publishing Group Inc.

Lakein, A. 1973. *How to Get Control of Your Time and Your Life*. New York: Signet.

Landau, C., Cyr, M.G., and Moulton, A. 1994. *The Complete Book of Menopause*. New York: Perigee Health.

LeShan, E. 1993. *Grandparenting in a Changing World*. New York: Newmarket Press.

LeShan, E. 1990. *It's Better to Be Over the Hill Than Under It*. New York: Newmarket Press.

Lewis, R. 1995. *A New Look at Growing Older*. Newport Beach, CA: Southland Publishing Co.

Mason, J.L. 1988. *Stress Passages*. Berkeley, California: Celestial Arts.

Maximin, A. and Stevic-Rust, L. 1996. *The Stop Smoking Workbook: Your Guide to Healthy Quitting*. Oakland, CA: New Harbinger Publications, Inc.

McKay, M., Davis, M., and Fanning, P. 1995. *Messages: The Communication Skills Book*, second edition. Oakland, CA: New Harbinger Publications, Inc.

McKay, M., Davis, M., and Fanning, P. 1994. *Couple Skills*. Oakland, CA: New Harbinger Publications, Inc.

McKay, M., and Fanning, P. 1993. *Self-Esteem*, second edition. Oakland, CA: New Harbinger Publications, Inc.

McKay, M., Davis, M., and Fanning, P. 1981. *Thoughts & Feelings*. Oakland, CA: New Harbinger Publications, Inc.

Mooney, A.J., Eisenberg, A., and Eisenberg, H. 1992. *The Recovery Book*. New York: Workman Publishing.

Rogers, J. 1995. *You Can Stop Smoking*. New York: Pocket Books.

Scaf, M. 1987. *Intimate Partners: Patterns in Love and Marriage*. New York: Random House.

Simon, J. 1996. "Getting Older," *Journal of Psychiatric Annals*, Vol. 26, No. 1

Solomon, M. 1994. *Lean on Me, The Power of Positive Dependency in Intimate Relationships*. New York: Simon & Schuster.

Tannen, D. 1990. *You Just Don't Understand*. New York: Ballantine Books.

Tyler, V. 1994. *Herbs of Choice—The Therapeutic Use of Phytomedicinals*. Binghamton, NY: The Haworth Press, Inc.

Tyler, V. 1993. *The Honest Herbal—A Sensible Guide to the Use of Herbs and Related Remedies*, third edition. Binghamton, NY: The Haworth Press, Inc.

Witkin, G. 1991. *The Female Stress Syndrome—Revised and Expanded Edition*. New York: Newmarket Press.

Zilbergeld, B. 1992. *The New Male Sexuality*. New York: Bantam Books.

References

Alberti, R.E., and Emmons, M.L. 1994. *Your Perfect Right*. San Luis Obispo, CA: Impact Publishers.

American Cancer Society. 1995. *Journal of National Cancer Institute*, 87(7), pp. 5177-23.

American Psychiatric Association. 1994. *Diagnostic and Statistical Manual of Mental Disorders*, fourth revised edition, Washington, DC: The American Psychiatric Association.

Amsterdam, J. 1996. "Mood Disorders in Women: Proceedings of a Symposium." Beechwood, Ohio: Current Therapeutics, Inc. (a division of Wyeth-Ayerst Laboratories).

Bart, P.B. 1971. "Depression in Middle Aged Women," *Women in Sexist Society: Studies in Power and Powerlessness*, Gornick V., Moran B.K., eds., New York: Basic Books.

Blumenthal, S.J. "Improving Women's Mental and Physical Health: Federal Initiative and Programs," *Women's Health Care*.

Burns, D.D. 1990. *The Feeling Good Handbook*. New York: Penguin Group.

Cancer Facts, 1992. National Cancer Institute: Menopausal Hormone Replacement Therapy and Cancer Risk, November.

Cone, F.K. 1993. *Making Sense of Menopause*. New York: A Fireside Book, Simon & Schuster.

Colditz, G., et.al. 1995. "The Use of Estrogens and Progestins and the Risk of Breast Cancer in Postmenopausal Women," *New England Journal of Medicine*, Vol. 332, No. 24, pp. 1589-93.

Consumer Reports. 1995. "Herbal Roulette." Vol. 60, No. 11, pp. 698-705.

Crosignani, P.G., Harlan, W., Stamfer, M., and Weger, N. 1994. *Women's Health in Menopause.* The Netherlands: Kluwer Academic Press.

Cutler, W., and Garcia, C. 1983. *Menopause: A Guide for Women and the Men Who Love Them.* New York: W.W. Norton & Co.

Flint, M.1976."Cross-Cultural Factors that Affect Age of Menopause," Consensus on Menopause Research of the Proceedings of the First International Congress on Menopause, Baltimore: University Park.

Gitlin, M., and Pasnau, R. 1989. "Psychiatric Syndromes Linked to Reproductive Function in Women: A Review of Current Knowledge," *American Journal of Psychiatry*, 146:11. pp, 1413-1422.

Hales, D., and Hales, R.E. 1995. *Caring for the Mind.* New York: Bantam Books.

Harvard Health Letter. 1996. "Too Many Vitamins?" Vol. 23, No. 3, pp. 1-3.

Harvard Women's Health Watch. 1995. "Dietary Fiber." Vol. III, No. 1, pp. 2-3.

———. 1996. "Herbal Remedies." Vol. III, No. 6. Feb. 1996, pp 2-3.

———. 1996. "The New Dietary Guidelines." Vol. III, No. 6, p. 1.

Kupperman, H.S., Wetchler, B., and Blatt, M. 1959. "Contemporary Therapy of the Menopausal Syndrome," *Journal of the American Medical Association*, Vol. 171, No. 12, pp. 1627-1637.

Landau, C., Carol, C., Michele, G., and Moulton, A. 1994. *Complete Book of Menopause.* New York: Perigee Health.

Lark, S.M. 1992. *The Menopause Self-Help Book.* Berkeley, CA: Celestial Arts.

Lutter, J.M., Bertrand, M., Strom, S., and Grumstrup, K. 1993. "Menopause and Physical Activity: What Is the Relationship?" *Melpomene Journal*, Vol. 12, #1, pp. 14-23.

McKay, M., Davis, M., and Fanning, P. 1995. *Messages: The Communication Skills Book*, second edition. Oakland, CA: New Harbinger Publications, Inc.

McKinlay, J., McKinlay, S., and Brambilla, D. 1987. "Health Status and Utilization Behavior Associated with Menopause," *American Journal of Epidemiology*, Vol. 125, pp. 110-121.

McKinlay, J., McKinlay, S., and Brambilla, D. 1987. "The Relative Contributions of Endocrine Changes and Social Circumstances to Depression in Mid-Aged Women," *Journal of Health and Social Behavior*, Vol. 28, pp. 345-363.

Mishell, D., and Paganini-Hill, J. 1994. *Management of Common Problems in Gynecology.* Cambridge. Blackwell Scientific Publications.

Mortel, K.F., and Meyer, J.S. 1995. "Lack of Postmenopausal Estrogen Replacement Therapy and the Risk of Dementia," *Journal of Neuropsychiatry Clinical Neurosciences*, 7(3), pp. 334-7.

Novak, Emil, as quoted in Furman, C.S. 1995. *Turning Point, The Myths and Realities of Menopause*, New York: Oxford University Press.

Parry, B. 1992. "Reproductive-Related Depressions in Women: Phenomena of Hormonal Kindling." *Postpartum Psychiatric Illness: A Picture Puzzle*. Hamilton, H.A., Harberger, P.N. (eds). Philadelphia: Univ. of Penn. Press.

Perry, S., and O'Hanlan, K. 1992. *Natural Menopause: The Complete Guide to a Woman's Most Misunderstood Passage*. Reading, MA: Addison-Wesley.

Shapiro, S. 1995. *Talking with Patients*. Northvale, NJ: Jason Aronson, Inc.

Shaw, R. 1992. *Gynecology*. New York: Churchill Livingstone.

Stamper, M.J., et.al. 1991. "Postmenopausal Estrogen Therapy and Cardiovascular Disease: 10 Year Follow-up from the Nurses' Health Study," *New England Journal of Medicine*, 325:11, pp. 756-762.

Tannen, D. 1990. *You Just Don't Understand*. New York: Ballantine Books.

Troisi, R., et.al. 1995. "Menopause, Postmenopausal Estrogen Preparations, and the Risk of Adult-Onset Asthma," *American Journal of Respiratory Critical Care Medicine*, Vol. 152, pp. 1183-1188.

Tubesing, N.L., and Tubesing, D.A. 1994. *Structured Exercises in Stress Management*, volumes 1-5. Duluth, MN: Whole Person Associates.

Wharton, L. 1995. *Natural Women's Health*. Oakland, CA: New Harbinger Publications, Inc.

The Writing Group for the PEPI Study. 1996. "Effects of Hormone Replacement Therapy on Endometrial Histology in Postmenopausal Women," The Postmenopausal Estrogen/Progestin Interventions (PEPI Study), *JAMA*, Vol. 275, No. 5, pp. 370-375.

Wyeth-Ayerst Laboratories. 1995. *Welcome to Seasons, Introductory Issue*. Philadelphia, PA: Wyeth-Ayerst Laboratories

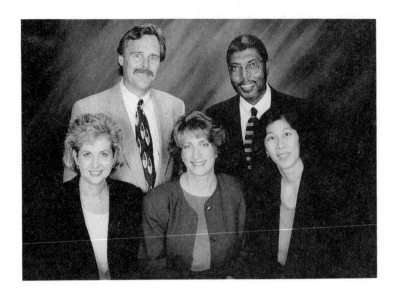

About the Authors

The authors are all on the board of directors of Pacific Mental Health Centers, based in Santa Clarita, California.

Robert M. Dosh, Ph.D., is a licensed psychologist in private practice and a licensed Marriage, Family, and Child Counselor. He specializes in the assessing and treating Attention Deficit Hyperactive Disorder in adults and children and in Tourette's Syndrome Disorder. Dr. Dosh lives in southern California with his wife and their two sons.

Susan N. Fukushima, M.D., is a board certified psychiatrist in private practice and an assistant clinical professor at UCLA Neuropsychiatric Institute. She specializes in the treatment of mood and anxiety disorders, PTSD, eating disorders, problems with relationships, and stress. Dr. Fukushima has written articles dealing with the treatment of rape victims and Asian Americans, and she has a longstanding interest in women's issues.

Jane E. Lewis, Ph.D., is a licensed psychologist and a licensed educational psychologist in private practice in Beverly Hills. In addition to her work as a specialist in psychological testing and evaluation, she also treats a wide range of psychological problems and disorders, including depression and relationship issues. Dr. Lewis lives in a beach community with her husband and two children.

Robert L. Ross, M.D., is a board certified psychiatrist and psychoanalyst practicing in Santa Monica, California, and an assistant professor of psychiatry at UCLA School of Medicine. A former epidemiologist intelligence services officer with the Centers for Disease Control and Prevention in Atlanta, Georgia, Dr. Ross's areas of interest are in cultural, racial, and gender issues as they affect personality development.

Lynne A. Steinman, Ph.D., is a licensed clinical psychologist in private practice. She specializes in stress management and anxiety, mood disorders, chronic illness and fibromyalgia, women's issues (including menopause), dementia, and caregiving. Dr. Steinman currently lives in Santa Clarita, California, with her husband and three dogs.

Other New Harbinger Self-Help Titles

PMS: Women Tell Women How to Control Premenstrual Syndrome, $13.95
Five Weeks to Healing Stress: The Wellness Option, $17.95
Choosing to Live: How to Defeat Suicide Through Cognitive Therapy, $12.95
Why Children Misbehave and What to Do About It, $14.95
Illuminating the Heart, $13.95
When Anger Hurts Your Kids, $12.95
The Addiction Workbook, $17.95
The Mother's Survival Guide to Recovery, $12.95
The Chronic Pain Control Workbook, Second Edition, $17.95
Fibromyalgia & Chronic Myofacial Pain Syndrome, $19.95
Diagnosis and Treatment of Sociopaths, $44.95
Flying Without Fear, $12.95
Kid Cooperation: How to Stop Yelling, Nagging & Pleading and Get Kids to Cooperate, $12.95
The Stop Smoking Workbook: Your Guide to Healthy Quitting, $17.95
Conquering Carpal Tunnel Syndrome and Other Repetitive Strain Injuries, $17.95
The Tao of Conversation, $12.95
Wellness at Work: Building Resilience to Job Stress, $17.95
What Your Doctor Can't Tell You About Cosmetic Surgery, $13.95
An End of Panic: Breakthrough Techniques for Overcoming Panic Disorder, $17.95
On the Client's Path: A Manual for the Practice of Solution-Focused Therapy, $39.95
Living Without Procrastination: How to Stop Postponing Your Life, $12.95
Goodbye Mother, Hello Woman: Reweaving the Daughter Mother Relationship, $14.95
Letting Go of Anger: The 10 Most Common Anger Styles and What to Do About Them, $12.95
Messages: The Communication Skills Workbook, Second Edition, $13.95
Coping With Chronic Fatigue Syndrome: Nine Things You Can Do, $12.95
The Anxiety & Phobia Workbook, Second Edition, $17.95
Thueson's Guide to Over-The-Counter Drugs, $13.95
Natural Women's Health: A Guide to Healthy Living for Women of Any Age, $13.95
I'd Rather Be Married: Finding Your Future Spouse, $13.95
The Relaxation & Stress Reduction Workbook, Fourth Edition, $17.95
Living Without Depression & Manic Depression: A Workbook for Maintaining Mood Stability, $17.95
Belonging: A Guide to Overcoming Loneliness, $13.95
Coping With Schizophrenia: A Guide For Families, $13.95
Visualization for Change, Second Edition, $13.95
Postpartum Survival Guide, $13.95
Angry All The Time: An Emergency Guide to Anger Control, $12.95
Couple Skills: Making Your Relationship Work, $13.95
Handbook of Clinical Psychopharmacology for Therapists, $39.95
The Warrior's Journey Home: Healing Men, Healing the Planet, $13.95
Weight Loss Through Persistence, $13.95
Post-Traumatic Stress Disorder: A Complete Treatment Guide, $39.95
Stepfamily Realities: How to Overcome Difficulties and Have a Happy Family, $13.95
Father-Son Healing: An Adult Son's Guide, $12.95
The Chemotherapy Survival Guide, $12.95
Your Family/Your Self: How to Analyze Your Family System, $12.95
Being a Man: A Guide to the New Masculinity, $12.95
The Deadly Diet, Second Edition: Recovering from Anorexia & Bulimia, $13.95
Last Touch: Preparing for a Parent's Death, $11.95
Consuming Passions: Help for Compulsive Shoppers, $11.95
Self-Esteem, Second Edition, $13.95
I Can't Get Over It, A Handbook for Trauma Survivors, 2nd Edition, $15.95
Concerned Intervention, When Your Loved One Won't Quit Alcohol or Drugs, $12.95
Dying of Embarrassment: Help for Social Anxiety and Social Phobia, $12.95
The Depression Workbook: Living With Depression and Manic Depression, $17.95
Focal Group Psychotherapy: For Mental Health Professionals, $44.95
Prisoners of Belief: Exposing & Changing Beliefs that Control Your Life, $12.95
Men & Grief: A Guide for Men Surviving the Death of a Loved One, $13.95
When the Bough Breaks: A Helping Guide for Parents of Sexually Abused Children, $11.95
Love Addiction: A Guide to Emotional Independence, $12.95
When Once Is Not Enough: Help for Obsessive Compulsives, $13.95
The Three Minute Meditator, 3rd Edition $12.95
Getting to Sleep, $12.95
Beyond Grief: A Guide for Recovering from the Death of a Loved One, $13.95
Leader's Guide to the Relaxation & Stress Reduction Workbook, Fourth Edition, $19.95
The Divorce Book, $13.95
Hypnosis for Change: A Manual of Proven Techniques, 3rd Edition, $13.95
When Anger Hurts, $13.95
Free of the Shadows: Recovering from Sexual Violence, $12.95
Lifetime Weight Control, $12.95

Call **toll free, 1-800-748-6273,** to order. Have your Visa or Mastercard number ready. Or send a check for the titles you want to New Harbinger Publications, 5674 Shattuck Ave., Oakland, CA 94609. Include $3.80 for the first book and 75¢ for each additional book to cover shipping and handling. (California residents please include appropriate sales tax.) Allow four to six weeks for delivery.

Prices subject to change without notice.